An Atlas of Histology

1. Haematoxylin and Eosin.

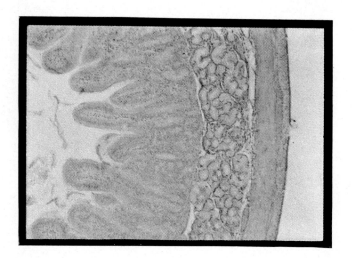

2. Haemalum, Van Gieson, and Alcian Blue.

3. Mallory triple stain, Azan.

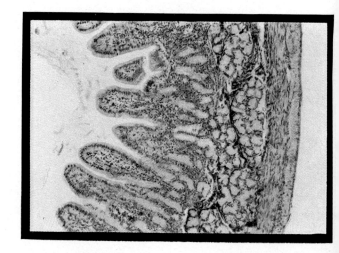

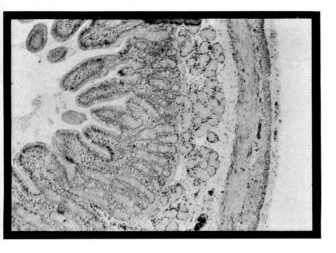

4. Iron Haematoxylin.

5. Periodic Acid—Schiff (P.A.S.).

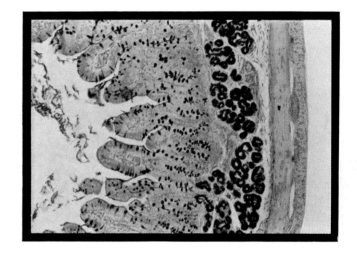

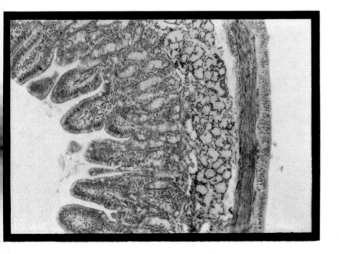

6. Masson Trichrome.

An Atlas of Histology

by the same authors
An Atlas of Embryology

an atlas of
HISTOLOGY

W. H. Freeman B.Sc. M.I.Biol.

Head of the Biology Department, Chislehurst and Sidcup Grammar School
Chief Examiner, 'A' Level Zoology, London

and

Brian Bracegirdle B.Sc. A.R.P.S. M.I.Biol.

Principal Lecturer in Science, College of All Saints, London
Assistant Examiner, 'A' level Zoology, London

Dover Publications, Inc. · New York

Book design by Alan Plummer

Published in the United States of America
by Dover Publications, Inc., New York
Printed in Great Britain by Bookprint Ltd

Preface

This book is designed to be an aid in the laboratory interpretation of histological preparations; except for a basic account of the tissues it does not seek to offer the theoretical background. The contents, selected to be of use for GCE 'A'-level and first degrees, represent the short version of a full atlas designed for second medical degree students. Our publishers have cooperated wholeheartedly in keeping the price at a level where the book is inexpensive enough for individual use.

All the photomicrographs and drawings have been made specially for the book, but without first class preparations our efforts would have been of no avail. Such preparations are made only by people who have devoted their lives to such work, and it has been our good fortune to receive wholehearted cooperation from many dedicated histologists whose slides made it possible for us to produce this work.

To Dr F. J. Aumonier of St Bartholomew's Medical College; Donald Canwell of the Physiological Laboratory, Cambridge; Professor Francis Davies of the Anatomy Department of the University of Sheffield; Professor Ben Dawes of King's College, London; the Biology Department of Goldsmiths' College, London; John Haller of Harris Biological Supplies Ltd; Professor W. J. Hamilton of Charing Cross Hospital Medical School, London; C. Heather of the Institute of Dermatology, London; John Kugler of the Department of Anatomy of the University of Sheffield; Dr Dennis Lacy of St Bartholomew's Medical College, London; Malcolm Scott of the Royal Veterinary College, London; Dr Gordon Thomas of Guy's Hospital Medical School, London; and Dr Graham Weddell of the Department of Human Anatomy of the University of Oxford, we owe our most sincere thanks for their generous help and advice.

To Professor Sir Bryan Matthews, C.B.E., F.R.S , of the Physiological Laboratory, Cambridge, we owe a special debt of gratitude for his early and continuing encouragement, and for his great courtesy in asking his chief technician, Donald Canwell, to give us every assistance. Mr Canwell proved to be our main support and so magnificent was his response that over half the preparations used by us were made by him, many specially.

Mr John Haller of Harris Biological Supplies has offered valuable comments and suggestions throughout, as well as providing many slides. It was as a result of Mr Haller's suggestion that this short version came to be written. His friend Mr Kugler, to whom he introduced us, has been a constant source of information, advice, and material; to both these gentlemen we are most deeply indebted.

Mr Malcolm Scott, our reader, has been a tower of strength. His suggestions on the text greatly improved it, and his care in checking all the labelling eliminated many errors. Any remaining are of course the sole responsibility of the authors.

We would also like to thank our layout artist, Mr Alan Plummer, for his skill and industry in the arrangement of the contents, and for designing the cover. In our publishers we have always found enthusiastic support and facilitation of our aims; particularly, Mr Hamish MacGibbon has cheerfully met all the many demands we have made upon him. Finally, we thank our wives for their continuing help and good humour in the face of the intense activity which took over so much of their homes so often.

March 1966   W.H.F.
                                                             B.B.

* Preparations marked with an asterisk in the list of contents are available as 2 x 2 colour slides for projection from *Philip Harris Ltd, 63 Ludgate Hill, Birmingham 3., England*

They are made from originals supplied by the authors exclusively to this company, and are recommended for their quality and moderate cost as excellent aids to the teaching of histology especially in conjunction with this book.

CONTENTS

TISSUES

THE UROGENITAL SYSTEM

THE SKIN

THE RESPIRATORY SYSTEM

THE NEUROSENSORY SYSTEM

THE SPINAL CORD

THE BRAIN

THE ENDOCRINE SYSTEM

THE CIRCULATORY SYSTEM

ORGAN RELATIONSHIPS

MITOSIS

INDEX

TISSUES

CELLS

Cells are units of protoplasm surrounded by a plasma membrane. They vary in diameter from 7.5μ (erythrocytes of man) to 85mm (ostrich egg). Usually each cell has a single nucleus separated from the cytoplasm by a perforated nuclear membrane: however, mammalian erythrocytes have no nuclei, while liver cells sometimes have two nuclei and osteoclasts seven or more. Cells are the functional units of the body capable of assimilating food, growing, respiring, excreting, secreting, responding to stimuli, and reproducing, though one or more of these functions may be lost in specialized cells. These activities depend upon cytoplasmic structures known as organelles.

The organelles of the cytoplasm are the endoplasmic reticulum, mitochondria, the Golgi apparatus, centrioles, ribosomes, and lysosomes. Non-living inclusions may occur in the cytoplasm – e.g. starch granules and fat droplets. Non-living material may also be produced outside cells – e.g. collagenous fibres and the matrix of bone.

The nuclei of cells stain darkly with haematoxylin and other basic dyes, whereas the cytoplasm stains with eosin, but there is no one staining technique which will demonstrate all cell components. The frontispiece shows the appearance of sections of duodenum stained by different techniques.

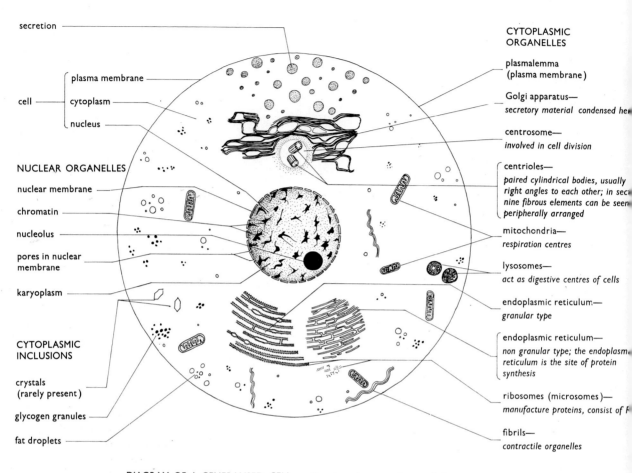

secretion

CYTOPLASMIC
ORGANELLES

cell — plasma membrane
cytoplasm
nucleus

plasmalemma
(plasma membrane)

Golgi apparatus—
secretory material condensed he▪

centrosome—
involved in cell division

NUCLEAR ORGANELLES

centrioles—
paired cylindrical bodies, usually
right angles to each other; in sec▪
nine fibrous elements can be seen
peripherally arranged

nuclear membrane

chromatin

nucleolus

pores in nuclear
membrane

mitochondria—
respiration centres

lysosomes—
act as digestive centres of cells

karyoplasm

endoplasmic reticulum—
granular type

CYTOPLASMIC
INCLUSIONS

endoplasmic reticulum—
non granular type; the endoplasm▪
reticulum is the site of protein
synthesis

crystals
(rarely present)

ribosomes (microsomes)—
manufacture proteins, consist of ▪

glycogen granules

fibrils—
contractile organelles

fat droplets

DIAGRAM OF A GENERALISED CELL   (based on electron micrographs)

TISSUES

A fertilized egg divides to form several smaller cells which are very much alike. After they have undergone morphogenetic movements, these cells become arranged in three germ layers, the ectoderm, endoderm, and mesoderm. The cells of each layer then differentiate along divergent lines to produce the tissues of the body.

A simple tissue may be defined as a group of cells of common origin having the same specialized structure which fits them to perform a common function. Such a simple tissue is, however, uncommon apart from epithelia, and most tissues are complex, being made up of several different kinds of cells. Tissues are the building blocks that form the organs. A sound knowledge of the tissues is therefore essential before an attempt can be made to study the structure of organs.

There are four categories of tissue:

epithelial tissue – derived from all three germ layers
connective tissue – derived from mesoderm
muscular tissue – derived from mesoderm
nervous tissue – derived from ectoderm.

EPITHELIAL TISSUE

There are two types of epithelia: A – covering epithelia, and B – glandular epithelia.

A. COVERING EPITHELIA

1. The cells form a continuous layer covering an internal or external surface.

2. The cells are held together at their common boundaries by a thin layer of intercellular substance.

3. One surface of each cell is free and often highly specialized.

4. The opposite surface rests on a basement membrane derived from the underlying connective tissue.

5. Blood vessels are absent.

6. Covering epithelia are exposed to physical injury and infection and act as protective layers.

7. Damaged cells are replaced by new ones and mitotic figures are common.

8. All the vital traffic of the body passes through epithelia – e.g. digested food, oxygen, waste products, secretions.

9. Some epithelia are specialized for the reception of stimuli.

Classification of Covering Epithelia

Covering epithelia are classified according to either the arrangement or the shape of the constituent cells.

CLASSIFICATION BASED ON CELL ARRANGEMENT

1. Simple epithelia – these are one cell thick.

2. Pseudostratified epithelia – these appear to be more than one cell thick but all the cells rest on the basement membrane.

3. Stratified epithelia – these are many cells thick.

CLASSIFICATION BASED ON CELL SHAPES

1. Squamous epithelia – these are made up of flattened cells shaped like paving stones.

2. Cuboidal epithelia – are made of isodiametric cells.

3. Columnar epithelia – consist of cells which are taller than they are wide.

4. Transitional epithelia – these are made up of cells which change their shape when the epithelium is stretched.

There are twelve possible classes if these two schemes of classification are combined, but only eight of these occur.

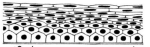

Simple squamous e.g. Bowman's
capsule of kidney

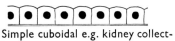

Simple cuboidal e.g. kidney collecting duct

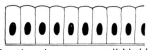

Simple columnar e.g. gall bladder

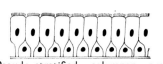

Stratified squamous e.g. oesophagus

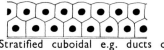

Stratified cuboidal e.g. ducts of
sweat glands

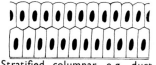

Stratified columnar e.g. duct of
mammary gland

Pseudo-stratified columnar e.g.
trachea

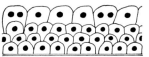

a) relaxed   Stratified transitional e.g. bladder   b) stretched

CLASSES OF COVERING EPITHELIA

B. GLANDULAR EPITHELIA

All living cells secrete and some, such as goblet cells, are highly specialized for this purpose. A gland is an organ largely composed of specialized secretory cells. The material secreted is usually a liquid containing such substances as enzymes, hormones, mucin, or fats.

Glands are epithelial in origin. The epithelial nature of the mucous membrane of the stomach is obvious. In most cases, however, the elaborate folding and branching of the invaginated epithelial layer that occur during development obscure the epithelial nature of glands.

Exocrine glands remain connected to a surface epithelium by the ducts through which they discharge their secretions. Endocrine glands, on the other hand, have no ducts and lose their epithelial connections. These ductless glands are highly vascular and discharge their secretions into blood vessels.

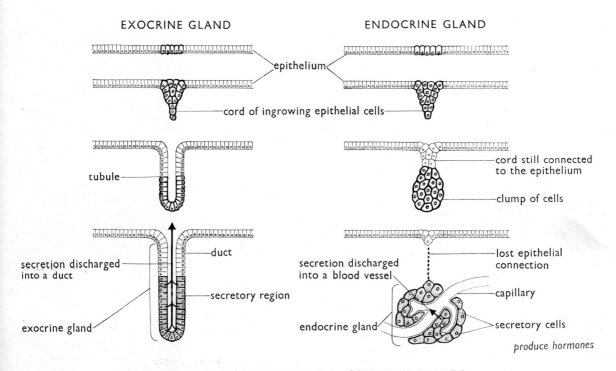

EXOCRINE GLAND   ENDOCRINE GLAND

epithelium

cord of ingrowing epithelial cells

tubule

cord still connected to the epithelium

clump of cells

duct

secretion discharged into a duct

secretory region

lost epithelial connection

secretion discharged into a blood vessel

capillary

exocrine gland

endocrine gland

secretory cells

produce hormones

DIAGRAM TO SHOW THE EPITHELIAL ORIGIN OF GLANDS

Secretions are produced by three distinct methods:

1. Merocrine. The secretion accumulates below the free surface of the cell through which it is released. There is no loss of cytoplasm. Merocrine secretion is exhibited by goblet cells and sweat glands.

2. Apocrine. The secretion accumulates below the free surface but can only be released by the breaking away of the distal part of the cell thus involving cytoplasmic loss. The mammary glands secrete milk in this manner.

3. Holocrine. The secretion is formed by the complete break-down of the secretory cells. Sebaceous glands are holocrine.

The ovary and testis are sometimes described as being cytogenous glands whose secretions are the germ cells.

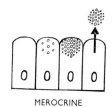

MEROCRINE

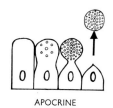

APOCRINE

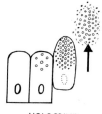

HOLOCRINE

DIAGRAM ILLUSTRATING SECRETION

Classification of Exocrine Glands

Glands are classified according to the shape of the secretory part (tubular or alveolar), and the nature of the ducts. If the duct is unbranched the gland is said to be simple; compound glands have branched ducts.

1. *Simple tubular*, e.g. crypt of Lieberkühn.

2. *Simple coiled tubular*, e.g. sweat gland.

3. *Simple branched tubular*, e.g. fundic gland (only the secretory part is branched).

4. *Simple alveolar*, e.g. mucous and poison glands in skin of frog (the term saccular is sometimes used for alveolar glands with a large lumen).

5. *Simple branched alveolar*, e.g. Meibomian gland (only the secretory part is branched).

6. *Compound tubular*, e.g. gland of Brunner (this is sometimes classified as a tubulo-alveolar gland since some secretory units are dilated).

7. *Compound alveolar*, e.g. lactating mammary gland.

8. *Compound tubulo-alveolar*, e.g. submaxillary gland.

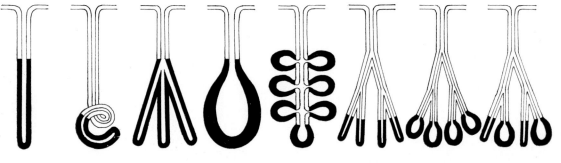

| Simple tubular | Simple coiled tubular | Simple branched tubular | Simple alveolar | Simple branched alveolar | Compound tubular | Compound alveolar | Compound tubulo-alveolar |

DIAGRAM TO ILLUSTRATE THE VARIOUS TYPES OF GLAND

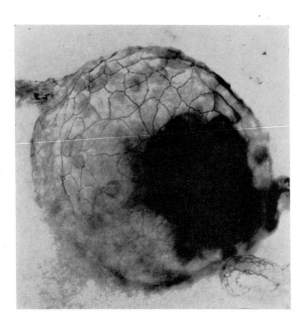

1. **Simple squamous epithelium,** surface view Bowman' capsule, (cat), mag. 350x

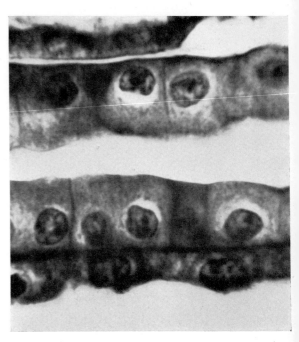

2. **Simple cuboidal epithelium,** L.S. kidney tubule, (monkey), mag. 1000x

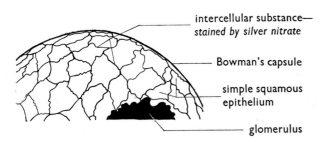

intercellular substance—
stained by silver nitrate

Bowman's capsule

simple squamous
epithelium

glomerulus

Drawing of specimen 1

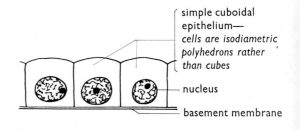

simple cuboidal
epithelium—
*cells are isodiametric
polyhedrons rather
than cubes*

nucleus

basement membrane

Drawing of specimen 2

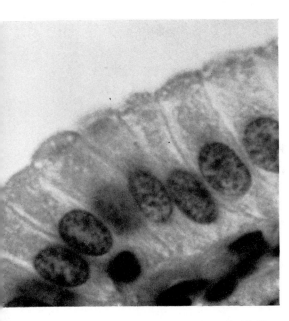

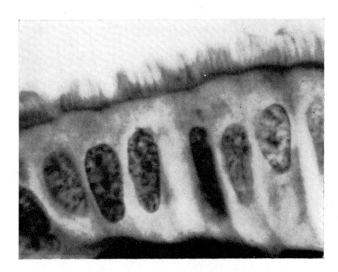

4. Simple ciliated columnar epithelium, T.S. oviduct, (rabbit), mag. 1000x

3. Simple columnar epithelium, L.S. gall bladder, (man), mag. 1150x

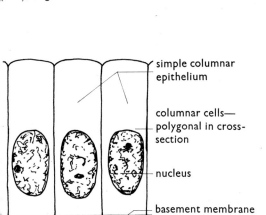

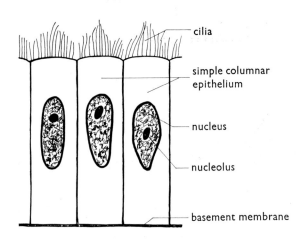

simple columnar epithelium

columnar cells—polygonal in cross-section

nucleus

basement membrane

Drawing of specimen 3

cilia

simple columnar epithelium

nucleus

nucleolus

basement membrane

Drawing of specimen 4

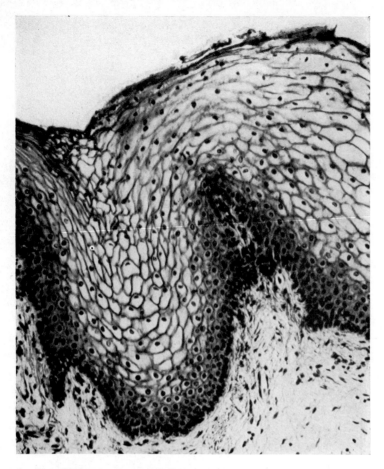

5. **Stratified squamous epithelium,** L.S. vagina, (man), mag. 200x

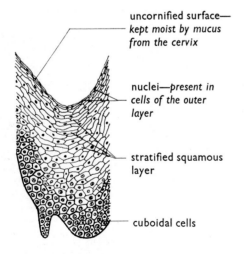

uncornified surface—
kept moist by mucus
from the cervix

nuclei—present in
cells of the outer
layer

stratified squamous
layer

cuboidal cells

Drawing of specimen 5

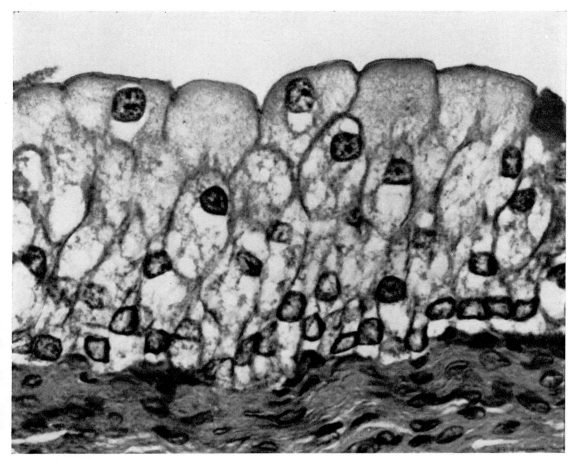

6. Transitional epithelium, relaxed V.S. bladder wall (rat), mag. 125x

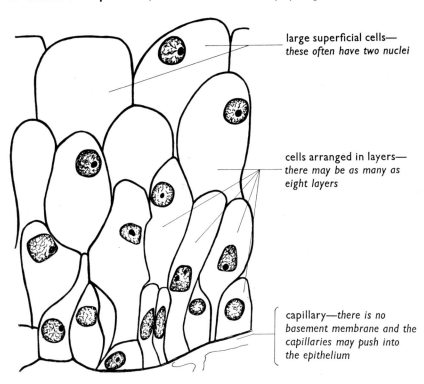

large superficial cells—
these often have two nuclei

cells arranged in layers—
*there may be as many as
eight layers*

capillary—*there is no
basement membrane and the
capillaries may push into
the epithelium*

Drawing of specimen 6

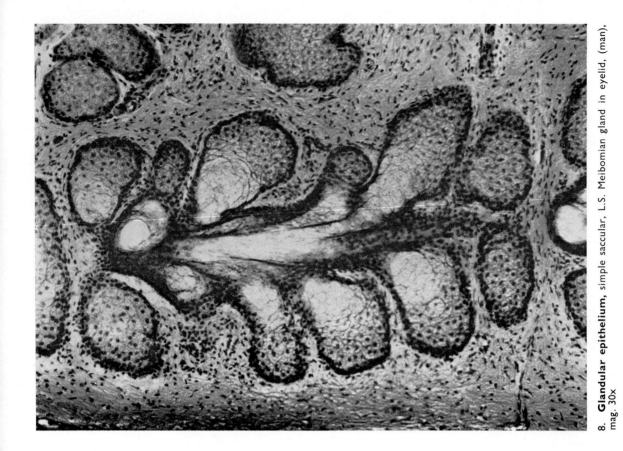

8. **Glandular epithelium,** simple saccular, L.S. Meibomian gland in eyelid, (man), mag. 30x

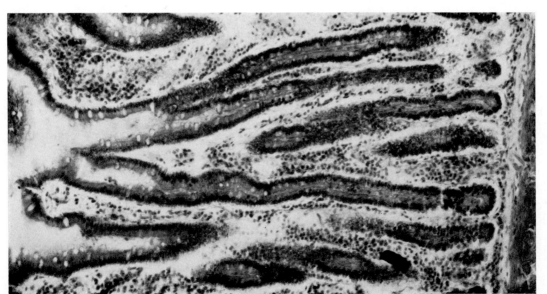

7. **Glandular epithelium,** simple tubular, VS. ileum, (man), mag. 85x

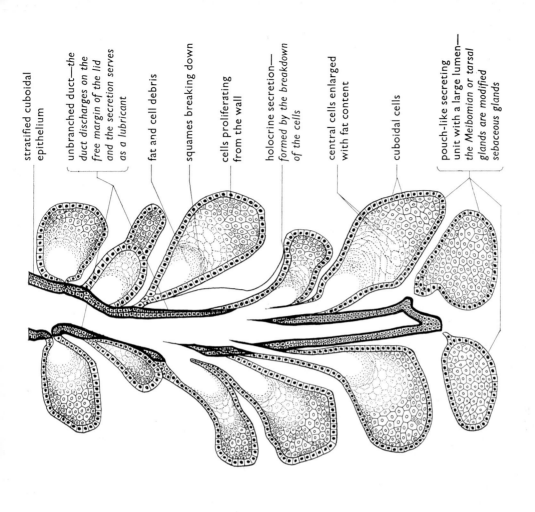

stratified cuboidal epithelium

unbranched duct—the duct discharges on the free margin of the lid and the secretion serves as a lubricant

fat and cell debris

squames breaking down

cells proliferating from the wall

holocrine secretion—formed by the breakdown of the cells

central cells enlarged with fat content

cuboidal cells

pouch-like secreting unit with a large lumen—the Meibomian or tarsal glands are modified sebaceous glands

Drawing of specimen 8

mocous membrane of ileum

space between villi—there are no ducts

simple columnar epithelium

two simple tubular glands—crypts of Lieberkühn

goblet cells

Paneth cells—zymogenic secretion of the merocrine type, i.e. the cells remain intact

Drawing of specimen 7

CONNECTIVE TISSUE

Early in the process of development stellate mesenchyme cells break away from the mesoderm, and these wandering cells become distributed between the three germ layers throughout the embryo. Connective tissue arises from these widely scattered free mesenchyme cells and is correspondingly ubiquitous in its distribution. Some of the mesenchyme cells remain in an undifferentiated condition in adult tissue.

Connective tissue is made up of cells, ground substance or matrix, and fibres. Matrix and fibres, which are non-living products of the cells, predominate, and form the supporting material of the body. As the name suggests, connective tissue serves as a connecting system binding all other tissues together.

Connective tissue forms sheaths around organs, bundles in which lie nerves and blood vessels, and sheets or fascia attaching the skin to underlying tissues.

The art of dissection is to display organs by separating them from their envelopes of obscuring connective tissue.

The sheaths around organs separate them from one another, enabling each organ to perform its special functions without interference from neighbouring organs. They also serve in defence against bacterial invasion, inflammation being an indication that a particular region has been invaded. Fat is stored in the superficial fascia, and this layer of adipose tissue provides insulation against heat losses from the skin. The skeletal framework of the body depends upon the specialized matrices of bone and cartilage for its rigidity.

Yet another kind of connective tissue, the haemopoietic tissue, is responsible for the production of blood cells.

The factor common to these diverse tissues is their origin from mesenchyme cells.

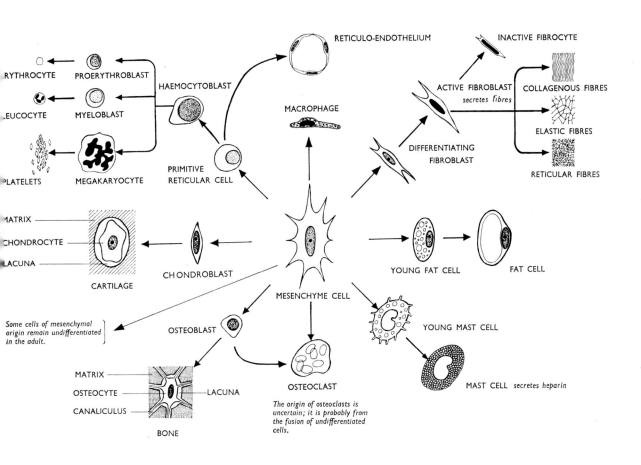

RETICULO-ENDOTHELIUM

INACTIVE FIBROCYTE

RYTHROCYTE   PROERYTHROBLAST

HAEMOCYTOBLAST

ACTIVE FIBROBLAST   COLLAGENOUS FIBRES
secretes fibres

MACROPHAGE

EUCOCYTE   MYELOBLAST

ELASTIC FIBRES

DIFFERENTIATING
FIBROBLAST

RETICULAR FIBRES

PLATELETS   MEGAKARYOCYTE

PRIMITIVE
RETICULAR CELL

MATRIX

CHONDROCYTE

LACUNA

CARTILAGE

CHONDROBLAST

MESENCHYME CELL

YOUNG FAT CELL   FAT CELL

*Some cells of mesenchymal
origin remain undifferentiated
in the adult.*

OSTEOBLAST

YOUNG MAST CELL

MATRIX

OSTEOCYTE

CANALICULUS

LACUNA

OSTEOCLAST

MAST CELL *secretes heparin*

*The origin of osteoclasts is
uncertain; it is probably from
the fusion of undifferentiated
cells.*

BONE

DIAGRAM ILLUSTRATING THE MAIN TYPES OF CONNECTIVE TISSUE CELLS
DERIVED FROM EMBRYONIC MESENCHYME

Classification of Connective Tissues

Connective tissues are classified according to the nature and arrangement of their non-living components. The classification below is based on that of Ham.

1. *Loose or areolar tissue.* A jelly-like ground substance containing cells and a loose network of fibres, e.g. in subcutaneous connective tissue.

2. *Adipose.* Similar to areolar tissue, but cells storing fat predominate, e.g. fat depots round the kidney.

3. *Dense fibrous.* Fibres predominate: a. regularly arranged, e.g. tendon, ligament, elastic ligament; b. irregularly arranged, e.g. dermis.

4. *Reticular.* A network of fine branching reticular fibres, which stain with silver, supporting parenchymal cells of viscera, e.g. spleen, liver.

5. *Cartilage.* A firm plastic matrix, containing fibres: a. Hyaline – translucent matrix with very fine collagen fibres, e.g. cartilage of trachea; b. Fibro-cartilage – dense collagenous fibres embedded in matrix, e.g. intervertebral disc; c. Elastic cartilage – elastic fibres embedded in matrix, e.g. cartilage of pinna, epiglottis.

6. *Bone.* Solid rigid matrix, containing collagenous fibres:
a. Spongy bone – trabeculae of bone between marrow-containing cavities, e.g. epiphysis of long bones, and inner regions of flat bones; b. Dense bone – formed of Haversian systems (osteones), e.g. shaft of long bones.

7. *Dentine.* Matrix similar to bone, e.g. teeth.

8. *Haemopoietic.* a. Myeloid, e.g. red marrow of ribs; b. Lymphatic, e.g. spleen, lymph nodes.

INTERCELLULAR SUBSTANCE

The following types of intercellular substance occur in connective tissue:

1. *amorphous ground substance*
2. *fibres: collagenous, elastic, reticular*
3. *matrix of cartilage, bone, dentine.*

Connective tissue cells depend on the diffusion of nutrient and waste materials in minute channels in bone and dentine, and through the amorphous matrix of all other connective tissues. Tissue fluid, an exudate of blood plasma, provides the medium for diffusion. An abnormal accumulation of this fluid occurs if its drainage into the lymphatic capillaries is impeded, resulting in the condition called oedema.

1. *Amorphous ground substance.* Composed of a mixture of muco-polysaccharides, e.g. hyaluronic acid and chondroitin sulphate with other unidentified substances.

Some bacteria invade connective tissue by secreting an enzyme, hyaluronidase, which digests the hyaluronic acid of the ground substance.

The amorphous material is metachromatic (i.e. it stains characteristically with toluidine blue and thionine, changing the colour of the stain), and gives a positive periodic acid Schiff reaction (i.e. carbohydrates present are oxidised by periodic acid to give aldehyde groups visualized with Schiff's reagent).

Basement membranes of epithelia are chemically similar to amorphous ground substance, and are PAS positive.

2. *Fibres.* Fibroblasts are connective tissue cells that secrete a fibre precursor which is condensed to collagen either within the cell or, more probably, on the cell surface. Fibroblasts are also thought to be responsible for the synthesis of elastic and reticular fibres and for the amorphous components of the intercellular substance.

CHART SUMMARISING THE PROPERTIES OF FIBRES

	COLLAGEN	ELASTIC	RETICULAR
appearance	colourless–hence known as white fibres	yellow – hence known as yellow fibres	only demonstrated by special silver techniques – hence called argyrophilic fibres
distribution	wide, particularly in tendon, joint capsules and ligaments	blood vessels, particularly aorta, lung, elastic ligaments, vocal cords	lymphatic system, particularly spleen; support basement membranes
structure	coarse; long fibres in wavy bundles; no branching; fibrils present	fine fibres which branch to form a network; no fibrils	fine short fibres which branch to form a close network; a few fibrils present
striations	electron micrographs reveal transverse striations, periodicity 640 A or 2,600 A	none	striations with periodicity of those of collagen fibres
tensile strength	great	little	little
elasticity	flexible but inelastic	considerable	little
refractive index	low	high	low
chemical composition	collagen, yields glycine on hydrolysis; boiling yields gelatin	elastin, yielding glycine and leucine on hydrolysis	reticulin, similar to collagen but exact nature unknown
pepsin digestion	rapid	resistant	
trypsin digestion	none	slow	none
weak acids and alkalis	cause swelling; dissolve	resistant	resistant
staining reactions:			
van Gieson	red	yellow	—
H. and E	pink	—	—
Mallory	blue	—	blue
Masson	green	—	green
resorcin fuchsin	—	dark purple	—
orcein	—	dark brown	—
silver	brown with some techniques	—	black

3. *Matrix.* The matrix of cartilage is composed of three substances:
  a. Chondromucoid – a glycoprotein
  b. Chrondroitin sulphate – strongly basophilic
  c. Albumoid – amount present increases with age.
The amorphous substance is permeated by fine collagenous fibres which are not visible in routine preparations.

The matrix of bone consists of a mineral component (about 65 per cent) and an organic component. The mineral matter is a compound of calcium and phosphate having the structure of a hydroxyapatite, $3Ca_3(PO_4)_2.Ca(OH)_2$. Some calcium carbonate is also present.

The organic matter is ossein which is very similar to collagen, yielding gelatin on boiling.

Dentine contains 70 per cent mineral matter and is similar to bone but harder. It is formed by odontoblasts; these cells send out slender processes which lie in the dentinal canals.

Transitional regions

Where two different types of connective tissue meet there is a transitional region at the junction where one type merges into the other, e.g. the insertion of tendons at a bony or cartilagenous surface.

Metaplasia

One type of connective tissue sometimes gives rise to another type, e.g. the pathological formation of nodules of bone in tendons. This is not due to conversion of tendon to bone. These metaplasia occur because the undifferentiated mesenchyme cells produce bone instead of tendon.

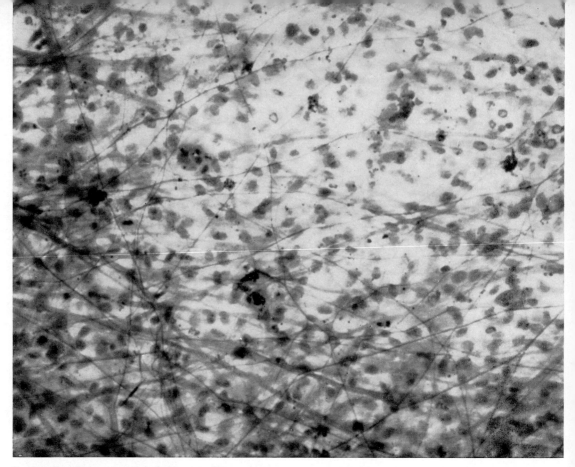

9. **Areolar tissue,** spread, (rabbit), mag. 420x

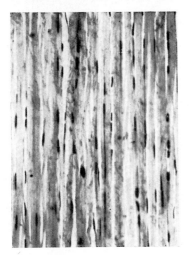

10. **Tendon,** L.S. (man), mag. 320x

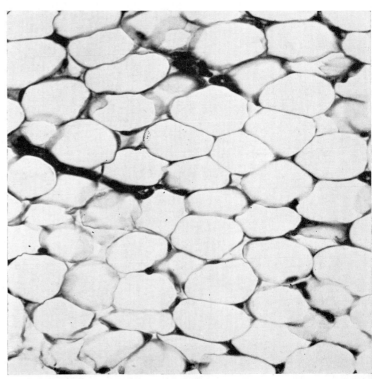

11. **Adipose tissue,** T.S. (cat), mag. 380x

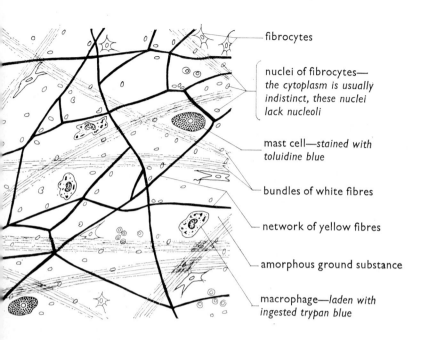

fibrocytes

nuclei of fibrocytes—
*the cytoplasm is usually
indistinct, these nuclei
lack nucleoli*

mast cell—*stained with
toluidine blue*

bundles of white fibres

network of yellow fibres

amorphous ground substance

macrophage—*laden with
ingested trypan blue*

rawing of specimen 9

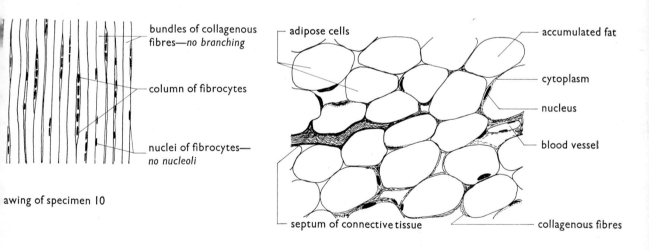

bundles of collagenous
fibres—*no branching*

column of fibrocytes

nuclei of fibrocytes—
no nucleoli

awing of specimen 10

adipose cells

accumulated fat

cytoplasm

nucleus

blood vessel

septum of connective tissue

collagenous fibres

Drawing of specimen 11

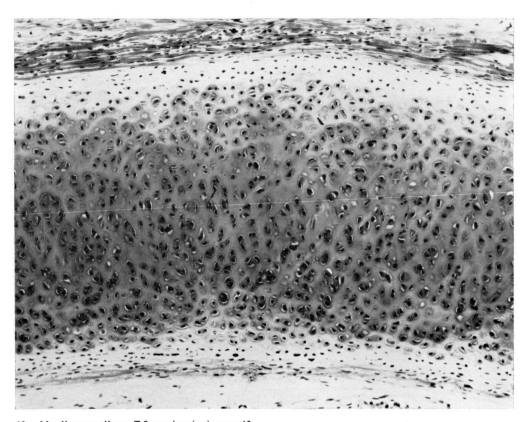

12. **Hyaline cartilage,** T.S. trachea (rat), mag. 60x

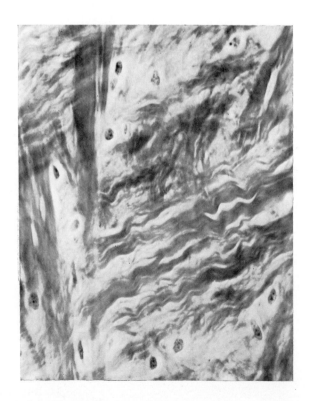

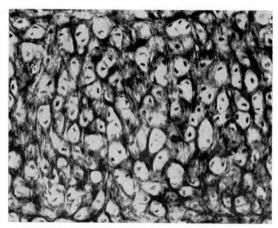

14. **Yellow elastic cartilage,** V.S. pinna, (man), mag. 75x

13. **White fibrous cartilage,** L.S. insertion of tendon on the patella (baboon), mag. 90x

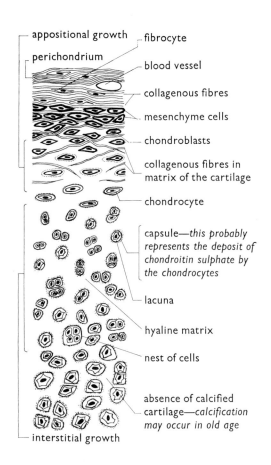

appositional growth
fibrocyte
perichondrium
blood vessel
collagenous fibres
mesenchyme cells
chondroblasts
collagenous fibres in matrix of the cartilage
chondrocyte
capsule—*this probably represents the deposit of chondroitin sulphate by the chondrocytes*
lacuna
hyaline matrix
nest of cells
absence of calcified cartilage—*calcification may occur in old age*
interstitial growth

Drawing of specimen 12

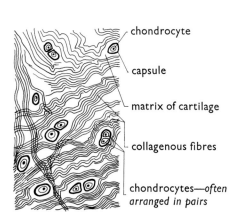

chondrocyte
capsule
matrix of cartilage
collagenous fibres
chondrocytes—*often arranged in pairs*

Drawing of specimen 13

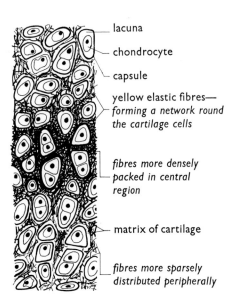

lacuna
chondrocyte
capsule
yellow elastic fibres— *forming a network round the cartilage cells*
fibres more densely packed in central region
matrix of cartilage
fibres more sparsely distributed peripherally

Drawing of specimen 14

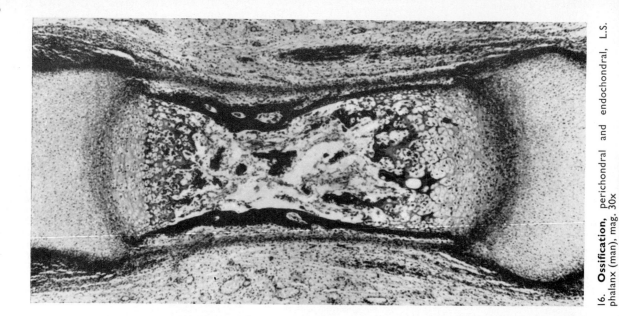

16. **Ossification,** perichondral and endochondral, L.S. phalanx (man), mag. 30x

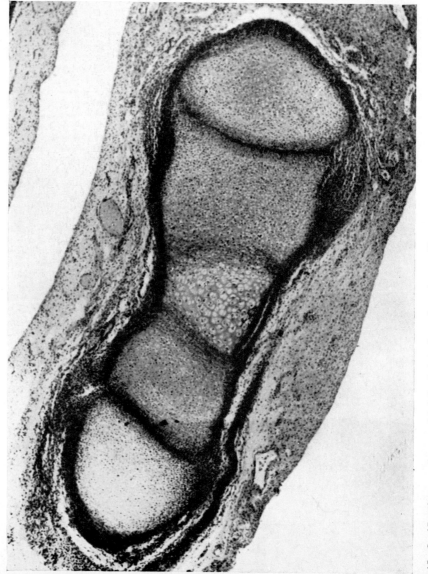

15. **Ossification,** cartilage model, L.S. phalanx (man, foetus), mag. 30x

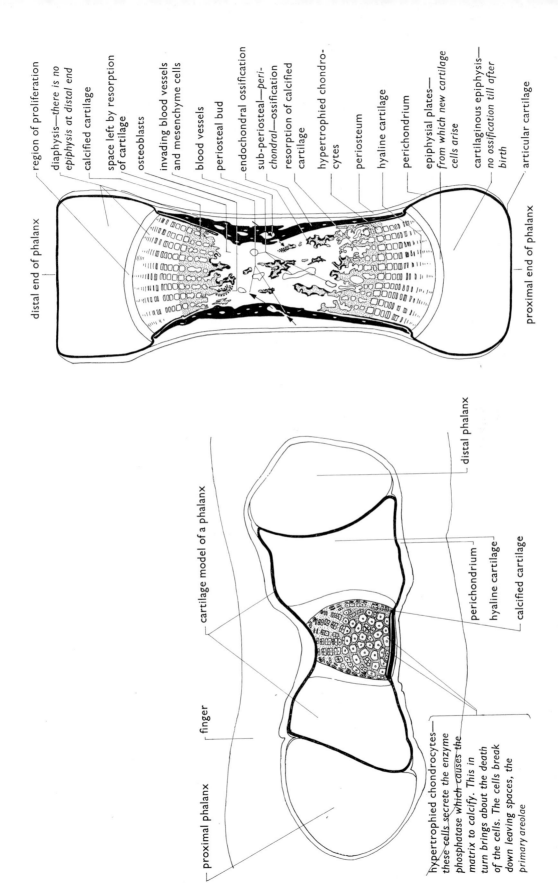

Drawing of specimen 16

region of proliferation

diaphysis—there is no epiphysis at distal end

calcified cartilage

space left by resorption of cartilage

osteoblasts

invading blood vessels and mesenchyme cells

blood vessels

periosteal bud

endochondral ossification

sub-periosteal—peri-chondral—ossification

resorption of calcified cartilage

hypertrophied chondro-cytes

periosteum

hyaline cartilage

perichondrium

epiphysial plates—from which new cartilage cells arise

cartilaginous epiphysis—no ossification till after birth

articular cartilage

distal end of phalanx

proximal end of phalanx

Drawing of specimen 15

cartilage model of a phalanx

distal phalanx

perichondrium

hyaline cartilage

calcified cartilage

finger

proximal phalanx

hypertrophied chondrocytes—these cells secrete the enzyme phosphatase which causes the matrix to calcify. This in turn brings about the death of the cells. The cells break down leaving spaces, the primary areolae

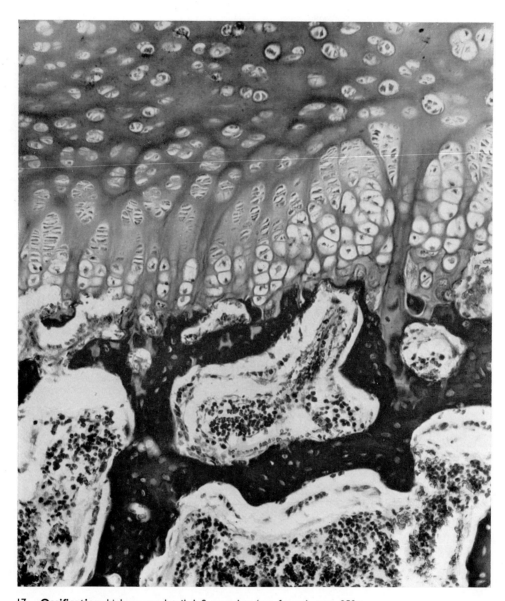

17. **Ossification,** high power detail, L.S. vertebra (rat, foetus), mag. 250x

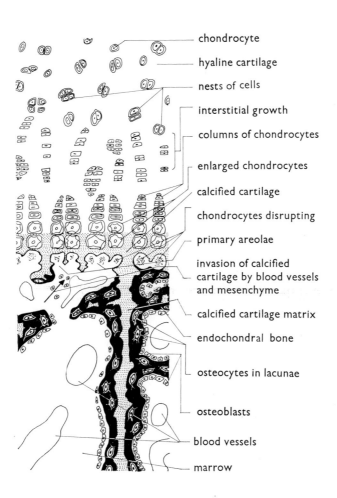

chondrocyte

hyaline cartilage

nests of cells

interstitial growth

columns of chondrocytes

enlarged chondrocytes

calcified cartilage

chondrocytes disrupting

primary areolae

invasion of calcified
cartilage by blood vessels
and mesenchyme

calcified cartilage matrix

endochondral bone

osteocytes in lacunae

osteoblasts

blood vessels

marrow

Drawing of specimen 17

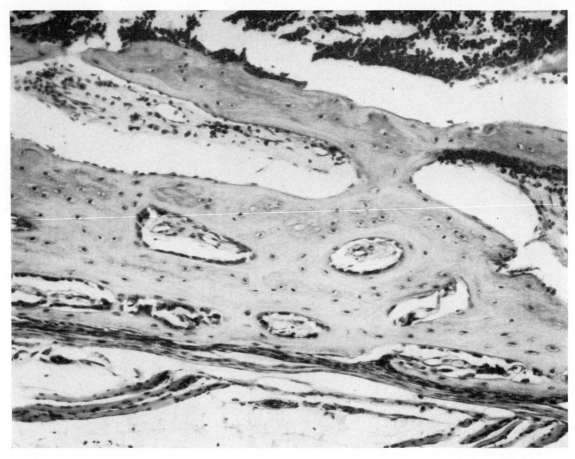

18. **Spongy bone,** L.S. femur (rat, foetus), mag. 120x

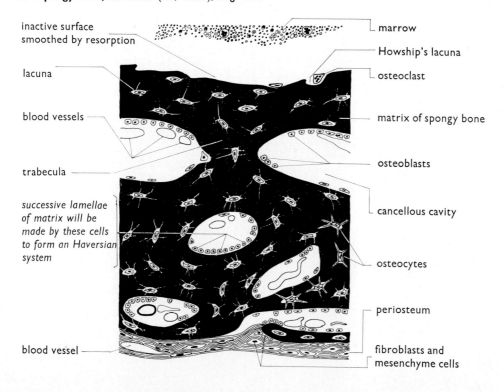

inactive surface smoothed by resorption

marrow

Howship's lacuna

lacuna

osteoclast

blood vessels

matrix of spongy bone

osteoblasts

trabecula

cancellous cavity

successive lamellae of matrix will be made by these cells to form an Haversian system

osteocytes

periosteum

blood vessel

fibroblasts and mesenchyme cells

Drawing of specimen 18

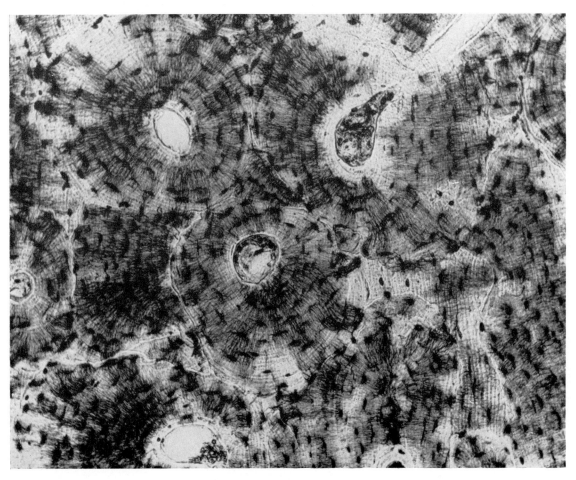

19. **Compact bone,** T.S. long bone ground (man), mag. 100x

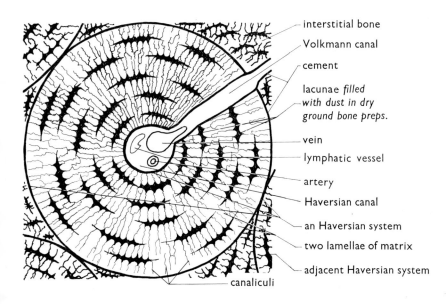

interstitial bone

Volkmann canal

cement

lacunae *filled with dust in dry ground bone preps.*

vein

lymphatic vessel

artery

Haversian canal

an Haversian system

two lamellae of matrix

adjacent Haversian system

canaliculi

Drawing of an Haversian system

MUSCULAR TISSUE

Muscular tissue is derived from mesoderm and is specialized for contraction. It is made up of elongated units, the muscle fibres, bound in a framework of vascular connective tissue which also provides an anchorage to the skeleton or skin.

Three different types of muscle fibre can be distinguished, each adapted to perform one special kind of contraction. Skeletal muscle contracts with rapidity during locomotion; the smooth muscle of the wall of the alimentary tract exhibits the slow rhythmic contractions of peristalsis; while the muscle of the heart continues to beat rhythmically, at a rate intermediate between that of skeletal and smooth muscle, throughout life.

The contraction of muscle fibres is brought about by a change in the arrangement of their protein molecules. The energy required is derived from the chemical energy of food.

Food and oxygen are supplied in blood circulating in an extensive network of capillaries within the muscle.

Striped muscle contracts in response to motor impulses from the central nervous system. Each motor nerve fibre has from ten to over one hundred branches each terminating at a motor end plate on a muscle fibre.

A motor axon, together with its end plates, constitutes a motor unit; the muscle fibres served by one motor unit contract in unison.

Information about the length of muscle tissue is relayed to the central nervous system, from muscle spindles, which act as stretch receptors.

The sensory input from muscle spindles modifies the outgoing motor impulses.

A CHART TO COMPARE THREE TYPES OF MUSCLE FIBRES

	SMOOTH	STRIPED	CARDIAC
pseudonyms	involuntary, non-striated, unstriped, plain	voluntary, striated, striped, red and white skeletal	heart
sarcolemma (shown by electron microscopy to be a composite structure)	absent	present. Consists of plasmalemma, basement membrane, and reticular fibres	present. Structure similar to that of striped muscle
myofibrils	inconspicuous	conspicuous	fairly conspicuous
length of fibre	0.02mm to 0.5mm	1 to 40mm	0.08mm or less
diameter of fibre	8 to 10μ at thickest part	10 to 40μ	15μ approx
branching of fibre	none	none	frequent
composition of fibre	single cell	multinucleate syncytium	single branching cell
nucleus	central	many nuclei at periphery of each fibre	central
cross striations	absent	present	present
intercalated discs	absent	absent	present
contraction	slow, rhythmic, sustained	rapid, powerful; not sustained	moderately rapid, with rests between contractions. Not sustained
control of contraction	impulses from CNS not essential for contraction	neurogenic; contracts only in response to motor impulses from CNS	myogenic; but rate controlled by autonomic nervous system
distribution	alimentary, respiratory, and urogenital tracts. Blood vessels and larger lymphatics. Main ducts of glands. Ciliary muscle of eye. Arrector pili muscle of skin	locomotory muscles. Sheets of muscle of abdominal wall etc. under skin. Diaphragm, middle ear muscles	heart only

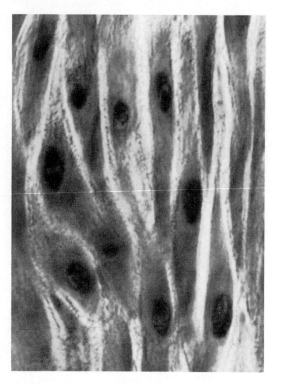

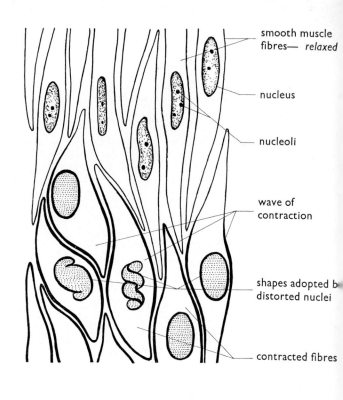

smooth muscle
fibres— *relaxed*

nucleus

nucleoli

wave of
contraction

shapes adopted b
distorted nuclei

contracted fibres

20. **Smooth muscle,** L.S. stomach, (rat), mag. 1100x

Drawing of specimen 20

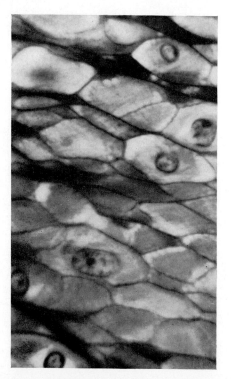

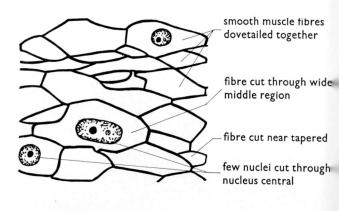

smooth muscle fibres
dovetailed together

fibre cut through wide
middle region

fibre cut near tapered

few nuclei cut through
nucleus central

21. **Smooth muscle,** T.S. duodenum,
(cat), mag. 1100x

Drawing of specimen 21

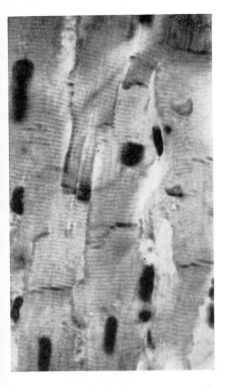

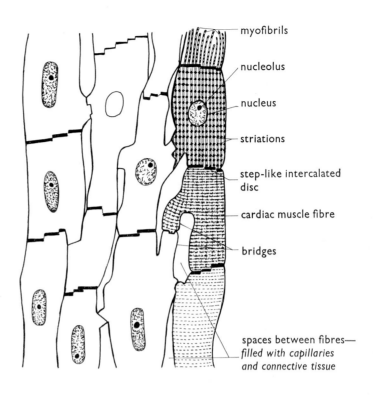

myofibrils

nucleolus

nucleus

striations

step-like intercalated
disc

cardiac muscle fibre

bridges

spaces between fibres—
*filled with capillaries
and connective tissue*

22. **Cardiac muscle.** L.S. ventricle, (man),
mag. 1100x

Drawing of specimen 22

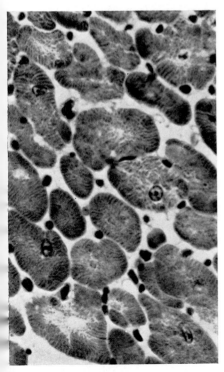

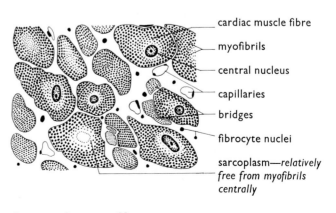

cardiac muscle fibre

myofibrils

central nucleus

capillaries

bridges

fibrocyte nuclei

sarcoplasm—*relatively
free from myofibrils
centrally*

23. **Cardiac muscle,** T.S. ventricle,
(sheep), mag. 110x

Drawing of specimen 23

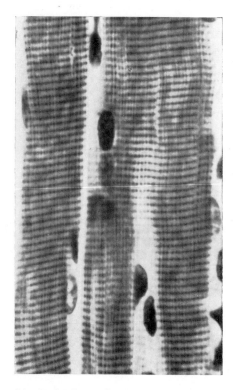

24. **Striped muscle,** L.S. rectus muscle of eye, (monkey), mag. 1100x

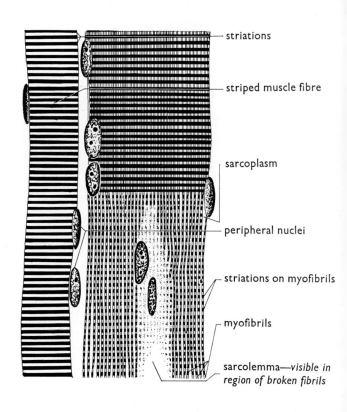

striations

striped muscle fibre

sarcoplasm

peripheral nuclei

striations on myofibrils

myofibrils

sarcolemma—*visible in region of broken fibrils*

Drawing of specimen 24

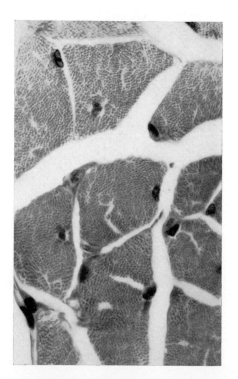

25. **Striped muscle,** T.S. rectus muscle of eye, (monkey), mag. 1100x

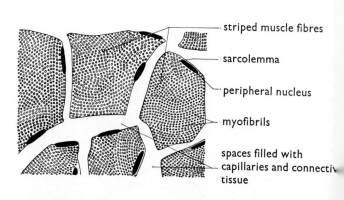

striped muscle fibres

sarcolemma

peripheral nucleus

myofibrils

spaces filled with capillaries and connectiv tissue

Drawing of specimen 25

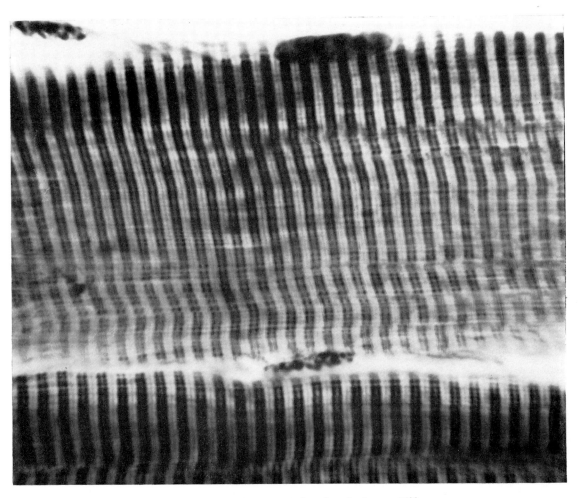

26. **Striped muscle**, L.S. rectus muscle of eye showing striations (monkey), mag. 2400x

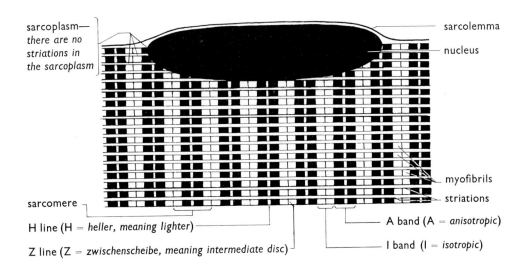

sarcoplasm— there are no striations in the sarcoplasm

sarcolemma

nucleus

myofibrils

striations

sarcomere

H line (H = *heller, meaning lighter*)

Z line (Z = *zwischenscheibe, meaning intermediate disc*)

A band (A = *anisotropic*)

I band (I = *isotropic*)

Diagram based on electron micrographs to explain specimen 26

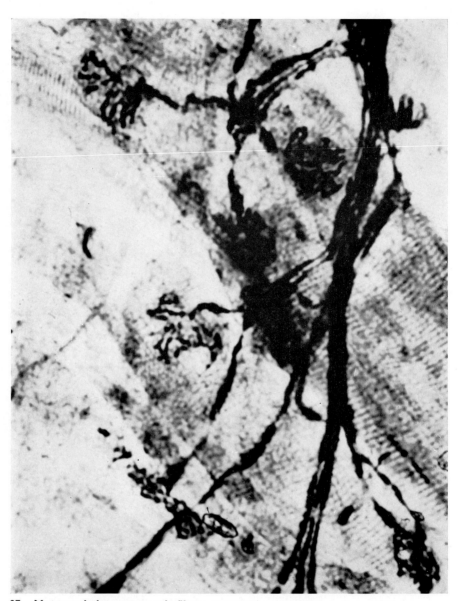

27. Motor end plates on muscle fibres, intercostal muscle squash (rat), mag. 800x

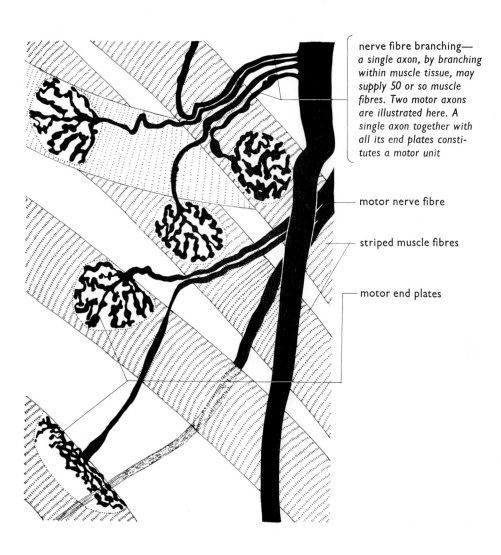

nerve fibre branching—
*a single axon, by branching
within muscle tissue, may
supply 50 or so muscle
fibres. Two motor axons
are illustrated here. A
single axon together with
all its end plates constitutes a motor unit*

motor nerve fibre

striped muscle fibres

motor end plates

Drawing of specimen 27

NERVOUS TISSUE

Nervous tissue develops from embryonic ectoderm. The unit of the nervous system is the nerve cell or neurone whose specialized cytoplasm is highly irritable and conductive. Neurones provide communication units linking receptors and effectors.

A nerve cell is irritable in the sense that it can be excited by a stimulus. A stimulus can be defined as a change in the intensity of applied physico-chemical energy acting in such a way as to tend to disturb the equilibrium of living protoplasm. The energy of the stimulus is transduced into electrical energy by neurones, and this electrical energy initiates a series of events which travel along the neurone. The wave of electrical change that is conducted constitutes a nerve impulse.

Neurones conduct nerve impulses either fully or not at all, and they are capable of conduction in either direction, but normally do so only in one direction. Afferent or sensory neurones conduct impulses towards the central nervous system, while efferent or motor neurones conduct away from it.

Neurones are specialized for conduction over long distances by having processes, which may be several metres long, extending from the cell body. A distinction may be made between processes called axons which normally conduct impulses away from the cell body, and dendrons which conduct towards it.

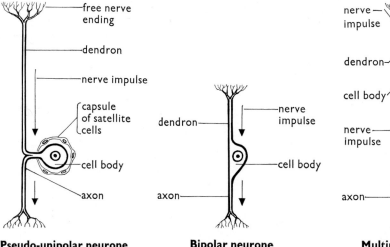

Pseudo-unipolar neurone
e.g. sensory neurone
of spinal reflex arc

Bipolar neurone
e.g. 2nd relay cell
of retina

Multipolar neurone
e.g. motor neurone
of spinal reflex arc

DIAGRAM ILLUSTRATING THE VARIOUS TYPES OF NEURONE

Nerve cells vary in the number of processes arising from them. Thus bipolar neurones have two processes while multipolar have many. A sensory neurone is described as pseudo-unipolar, since its single process is thought to consist of two closely opposed processes, although the evidence for this is not conclusive.

The processes of nerve cells are called nerve fibres. These occur in all parts of the nervous system. The white matter of brain and spinal cord is almost entirely nerve fibres; fibres are also profusely distributed throughout the grey matter. Nerves outside the central system are made up of nerve fibres supported by connective tissue.

Neurones are large cells. The nucleated part of the neurone is referred to as the cell body, the cytoplasm round the nucleus being called the perikaryon. The large spherical nucleus stains palely, but a conspicuous deeply staining nucleolus is present.

Cell bodies occur mainly in the grey matter of the central nervous system and in ganglia. Within the cytoplasm of the neurone are delicate threads, the neurofibrils, extending from the cell body into the processes. They are demonstrated by silver techniques. Varying amounts of granular chromophil material occur in the cytoplasm; this material forms Nissl's granules, which stain with toluidine blue and thionine. Nissl's granules consist of ribonucleoprotein, and are associated with protein synthesis. They extend into the dendrons but are absent from the axon hillock.

All neurones contain a reticular Golgi apparatus, but lack a centrosome. Once a nerve cell has differentiated, it loses the ability to divide; this may be related to the absence of a centrosome. Pigment granules of melanin and lipochrome are often present in neurones.

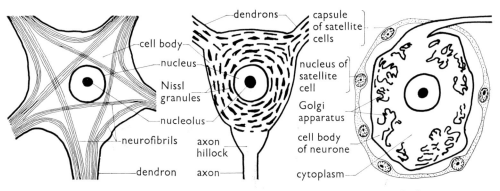

nerve cell body in a silver preparation of spinal cord of pigeon showing neurofibrils

motor neurone in a methylene blue preparation of spinal cord of cat showing Nissl granules

pseudo-unipolar neurone in a silver preparation of the dorsal root ganglion showing the Golgi apparatus

DIAGRAM TO ILLUSTRATE THE DETAILED STRUCTURE OF THE CELL BODY OF NEURONES

Nerve cells have associated with them another remarkable kind of cell, the Schwann cells. The relationship is an intimate one in which the nerve fibres are enclosed within folds of the Schwann cells. These are arranged along the length of nerve fibres, the gaps between successive cells being the nodes of Ranvier seen in medullated nerve fibres. There are no nodes in non-medullated fibres, and the nerves differ also in the number of fibres enclosed by a Schwann cell. In non-medullated nerves, as many as nine nerve fibres may be enfolded by each Schwann cell; in medullated nerves the Schwann cell wraps round a single fibre. The elaborate coiling of the Schwann cells round medullated fibres can be seen only in electron micrographs.

Schwann cells are rich in fat, hence the medullary sheath which they form appears as a dark ring round transversely cut fibres in osmic preparations.

Nerve fibres are of different diameters, and there is close correlation between thickness of fibre and speed of conduction; thick fibres conducting faster than thin. Erlanger and Gasser describe the following categories: 'A' fibres are up to 20μ in diameter. Their conduction velocities range from 90 metres/second to 2 metres/second. This group may be subdivided into categories according to the size of the action potentials. Medullated fibres of peripheral nerves belong to this group. 'B' fibres are from 1 to 5μ thick. Their conduction velocities are from 14 to 2 metres/second. The fine medullated preganglionic fibres of white rami belong to this group. 'C' fibres are from 0.4 to 1.0μ thick, and their conduction velocity is about 1 metre/second. This group includes some sensory fibres and non-medullated post-ganglionic fibres.

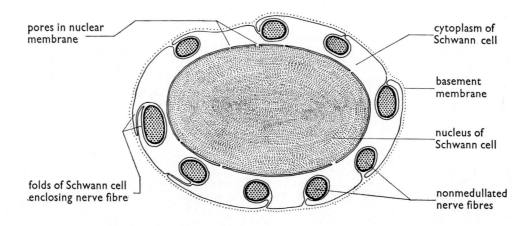

pores in nuclear membrane

cytoplasm of Schwann cell

basement membrane

nucleus of Schwann cell

folds of Schwann cell enclosing nerve fibre

nonmedullated nerve fibres

DRAWING OF NONMEDULLATED FIBRES   (from an electron micrograph)

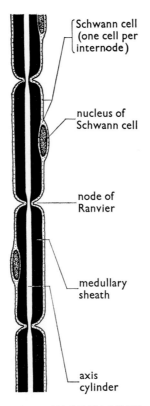

Schwann cell (one cell per internode)

nucleus of Schwann cell

node of Ranvier

medullary sheath

axis cylinder

DIAGRAM OF AN OSMIC
PREPARATION OF A
MEDULLATED NERVE FIBRE

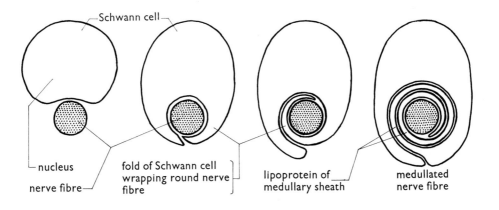

Schwann cell

nucleus

nerve fibre

fold of Schwann cell wrapping round nerve fibre

lipoprotein of medullary sheath

medullated nerve fibre

DIAGRAM TO SHOW THE FORMATION OF THE MEDULLARY SHEATH

At its termination each nerve fibre, whether axon or dendron, has a specialized nerve ending. There are three types of these:

a. Sensory – these terminate sensory dendrons, and are specialized for the reception of stimuli. The endings may be naked, as with free nerve endings, or encapsulated as in a tactile (Meissner's) corpuscle. b. Motor. Motor axons terminate in effectors such as muscles and glands. Motor end plates are the nerve endings of motor axons in muscle fibres. c. Synapses. Every nerve cell has at least one of its sets of nerve endings associated with another nerve cell; all the nerve endings of association neurones are associated with other neurones. The region where the nerve endings of one cell come into contact with another cell is known as the synapse.

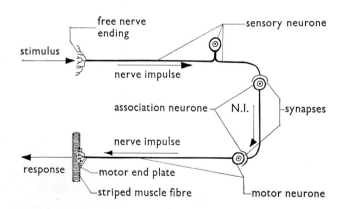

DIAGRAM TO SHOW THE RELATIONSHIP BETWEEN NEURONES

The synapse.

Within the central nervous system and ganglia, each axon breaks up into fine branches with terminal swellings. These are called end-bulbs, end-feet, or boutons terminaux, and they rest on the surface of the cell body and the dendrons of the neurone with which they have a synaptic relationship. Each neurone has synaptic relationships with axons from many other neurones.

The cytoplasm of the end-bulb and of the cell body with which it forms a synapse is rich in mitochrondria; the end-bulb is in all probability a region of great metabolic activity. When a nerve impulse reaches an end-foot it can go no farther, but must excite the next neurone to conduct. This excitation is effected by the secretion of a transmitted substance from the end-feet. Transmitter substance then diffuses across the synaptic gap into the adjacent cell, which is excited to activity, thereby effecting the relay of an impulse from one neurone to the next. The transneural relay at a synapse is in one direction only.

Acetylcholine and noradrenaline have been identified as transmitter substances. Fibres, such as those of the parasympathetic system, which secrete acetylcholine are said to be cholinergic, whereas postganglionic sympathetic fibres, which secrete noradrenaline, are said to be adrenergic.

When a nerve fibre degenerates its end-bulbs exhibit characteristic changes, becoming hollow and dilated. Use has been made of these changes in locating the synaptic relationships of nerve fibres: after a group of fibres has been severed experimentally, their synaptic endings can be identified in sections by their large hollow end-bulbs.

Nerve fibres that have been cut experimentally or have degenerated pathologically can only regenerate from the cell body.

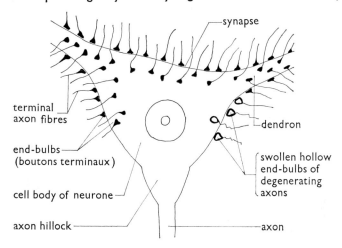

DIAGRAM TO SHOW SYNAPSES

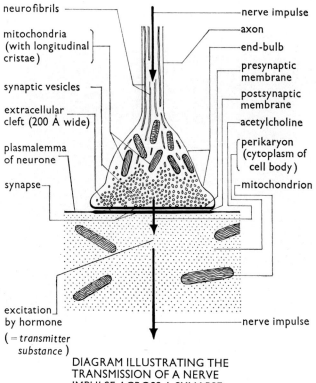

neurofibrils —————————————— nerve impulse

mitochondria } ————————————— axon
(with longitudinal
cristae) } —————————————— end-bulb

—————————————————— presynaptic
membrane

synaptic vesicles ———————————— postsynaptic
membrane

extracellular ——————————————— acetylcholine
cleft (200 Å wide)

———————————————————— perikaryon
(cytoplasm of
cell body)

plasmalemma ———————————————— mitochondrion
of neurone

synapse —

excitation —
by hormone —————————————————— nerve impulse

(= transmitter
substance)

DIAGRAM ILLUSTRATING THE
TRANSMISSION OF A NERVE
IMPULSE ACROSS A SYNAPSE

Neuroglia

This term is applied to cells other than neurones occurring in the central nervous system. Included in this category are the ependyma cells which line the cavities of brain and spinal cord; these cells are ciliated in the embryo. Among the 'glia' cells are the astrocytes, oligodendrocytes, and microglia. Fibrous astrocytes have feet resting on blood vessels and probably serve as supply routes conveying nutrients from the blood to neurones.

There are ten times more neuroglia cells than neurones in the brain, occupying half the volume. The metabolism of glia cells, RNA synthesis in particular, is closely linked to that of the neurones they surround. Possibly giant RNA molecules play an important part in memory, providing a biochemical means of storing coded information.

NEUROGLIA

Oligodendroglia

Microglia

Protoplasmic astrocyte

Embryo　Adult

Ependymal cells

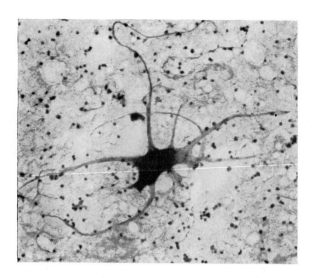

28. **Multipolar neurone,** brain smear (cat), mag. 140x

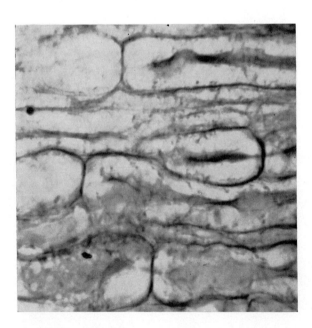

29. **Nodes of Ranvier,** L.S. posterior root nerve (cat), mag. 950x

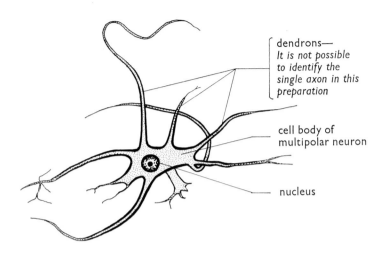

dendrons—
*It is not possible
to identify the
single axon in this
preparation*

cell body of
multipolar neuron

nucleus

Drawing of specimen 28

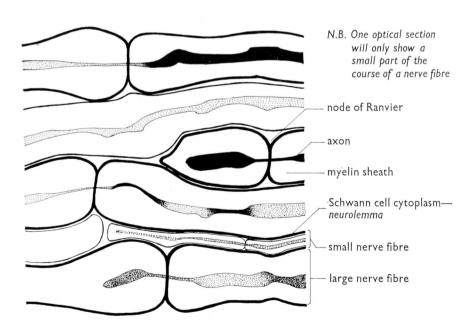

*N.B. One optical section
will only show a
small part of the
course of a nerve fibre*

node of Ranvier

axon

myelin sheath

Schwann cell cytoplasm—
neurolemma

small nerve fibre

large nerve fibre

Drawing of specimen 29

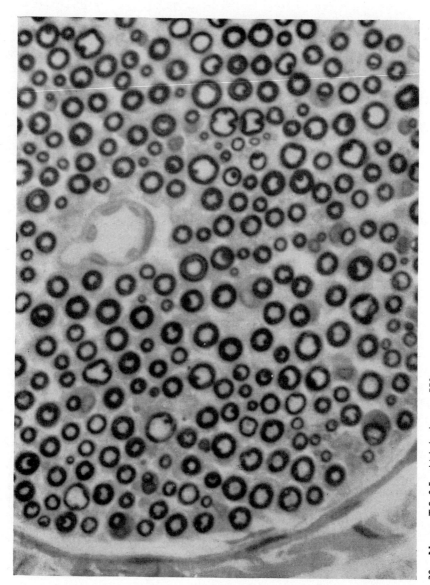

30. **Nerve**, T.S. 0.5u thick (rat), mag. 550x

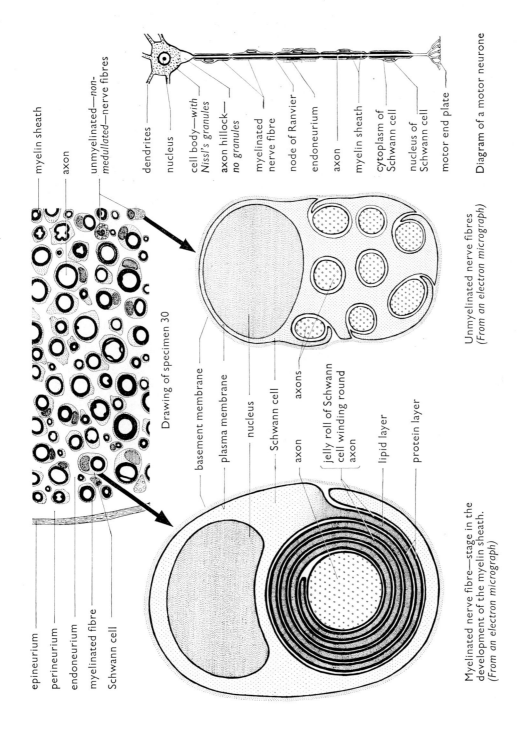

myelin sheath

axon

unmyelinated—non-
medullated—nerve fibres

dendrites

nucleus

cell body—with
Nissl's granules

axon hillock
no granules

myelinated
nerve fibre

node of Ranvier

endoneurium

axon

myelin sheath

cytoplasm of
Schwann cell

nucleus of
Schwann cell

motor end plate

Diagram of a motor neurone

epineurium

perineurium

endoneurium

myelinated fibre

Schwann cell

Drawing of specimen 30

basement membrane

plasma membrane

nucleus

Schwann cell

axon

axons

Unmyelinated nerve fibres
(From an electron micrograph)

jelly roll of Schwann
cell winding round
axon

lipid layer

protein layer

Myelinated nerve fibre—stage in the
development of the myelin sheath.
(From an electron micrograph)

ORGANS

THE DIGESTIVE SYSTEM

The digestive tract is in a sense external to the other systems, its lumen being continuous with the outside world. The lining of the tract acts in a defensive capacity. Before food can be used by the body it has to undergo mechanical and chemical changes. These changes are accomplished, stage by stage, in the various regions of the system, starting with mechanical breakdown by teeth and tongue in the buccal cavity. Food is moved from region to region by peristaltic waves of contraction of the smooth muscle fibres in the wall of the gut tube. The smooth muscle layer also provides a churning action which mixes the food with digestive juices. The chemical changes are hydrolytic and are catalysed by enzymes. The necessary water for hydrolysis is provided by copious secretion from the lining epithelium and glands of the gut. Mucus assists movement by acting as a lubricant. Digestive enzymes are secreted by glands either in the gut wall, e.g. glands of the stomach, or outside the tract, e.g. pancreas, in which case the secretion is poured into the gut along ducts.

The products of digestion, mainly soluble substances, are absorbed through the villi of the small intestine. The remaining water is absorbed principally through the wall of the large intestine.

Each region of the alimentary canal is adapted to its special functions. The special features of the regions are listed in the accompanying table. Histologically all regions exhibit a common basic plan which is illustrated in the diagram.

GENERAL HISTOLOGY OF THE ALIMENTARY CANAL

The alimentary canal may be identified by its tubular nature and the division of its wall into four distinct layers, namely:

1. *Mucosa*
2. *Submucosa*
3. *Muscularis externa*
4. *Serosa*

1. *Mucosa*. This is the innermost layer of the alimentary canal, consisting of three layers.

a. Epithelium. This layer is derived from embryonic endoderm except for the anal canal and part of the buccal cavity which are ectodermal in origin (the other layers of the wall are of mesodermal origin). All the glands of the digestive system develop from this epithelium.

b. Lamina propria. This is a layer of loose connective tissue which supports the epithelium. In most regions the lamina propria accommodates glands; it also contains blood vessels, lymphatic vessels, and may contain lymph nodes.

c. Muscularis mucosa. This constitutes the outermost layer of the mucosa; it is made up of smooth muscle fibres.

2. *Submucosa*. This is largely composed of collagenous fibres but elastic fibres are also present. The submucosa accommodates blood vessels, lymphatic vessels, nerves, and Meissner's plexus. Glands occur in the submucosa of the oesophagus and duodenum. Lymphatic tissue projects into the submucosa, particularly in the large intestine.

3. *Muscularis externa*. In most regions this is made up of an outer sheet of longitudinally arranged smooth muscle fibres and an inner sheet of circularly arranged fibres. Auerbach's plexus lies between these sheets of muscle fibres and co-ordinates their activities.

4. *Serosa*. This is a layer of areolar tissue continuous with the mesenteries supporting the gut.

DIGESTIVE SYSTEM

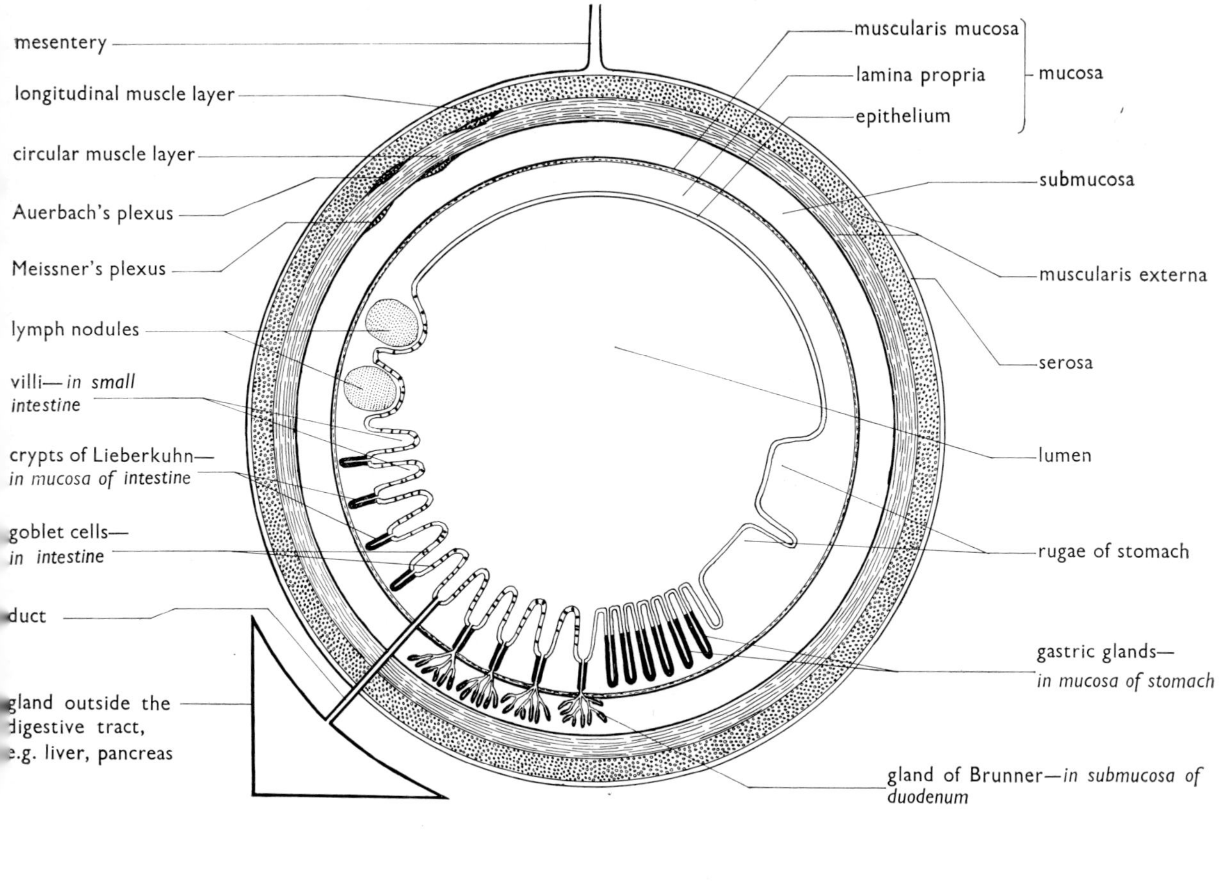

mesentery

longitudinal muscle layer

circular muscle layer

Auerbach's plexus

Meissner's plexus

lymph nodules

villi—*in small intestine*

crypts of Lieberkuhn— *in mucosa of intestine*

goblet cells— *in intestine*

duct

gland outside the digestive tract, e.g. liver, pancreas

muscularis mucosa

lamina propria — mucosa

epithelium

submucosa

muscularis externa

serosa

lumen

rugae of stomach

gastric glands— *in mucosa of stomach*

gland of Brunner—*in submucosa of duodenum*

DIAGRAM TO SHOW THE GENERAL PLAN OF THE ALIMENTARY CANAL

THE MAIN FEATURES OF THE ALIMENTARY CANAL

REGION	MUSCULARIS EXTERNA	SUBMUCOSA	MUSCULARIS MUCOSA	LAMINA PROPRIA	SURFACE EPITHELIUM	GLANDS	DIAGNOSTIC FEATURES
			MUCOSA				
OESOPHAGUS	Two layers, outer longitudinal and inner circular forming a thick muscular coat. In man, upper third has striped fibres, middle mixed, and lower third has smooth fibres.	Where muscularis mucosa absent it merges with lamina propria; elastic to allow for stretching during swallowing; contains mucous glands.	Thick; fibres longitudinally arranged. In man it is incomplete or absent from the upper third.	Rich in collagen fibres; has papillae projecting into epithelium; some glands occur here at either extremity of the oesophagus.	Stratified non-keratinised squamous type. In some mammals it is keratinised. Thrown into longitudinal folds reducing lumen to small star-shaped space.	Mucous glands in submucosa; some occur in lamina propria; few glands in man.	1. folded mucosa 2. stratified squamous epithelium 3. thick muscularis mucosa 4. absence of serosa 5. thickest muscularis externa 6. papillae project into epithelium
STOMACH	Three layers, outer longitudinal, middle circular, inner oblique. Oblique layer not continuous and is absent in pyloric region.	Forms large part of substance of folds (rugae).	Two layers; outer longitudinal and inner circular. Some fibres pass up between glands to be attached to epithelial basement membrane.	Loose connective tissue reduced in amount by closely-packed glands; contains some lymph nodules.	Simple columnar type; all cells alike, i.e. mucus-secreting. Gastric pits dip down to glands.	Fairly long and close together, confined to lamina propria. 3 types: 1. Cardiac, compound tubular, mucus secreting. 2. Fundic, simple branched tubular; chief, parietal, and mucous neck cells; secrete pepsinogen, rennin, mucus and HCl. 3. Pyloric; simple branched tubular; secrete mucus and possibly some enzymes.	1. rugae 2. thick wall 3. gastric pits 4. uniform epithelium 5. abundant glands in lamina propria 6. parietal cells in fundus 7. oblique layer in muscularis externa 8. no goblet cells 9. no villi
DUODENUM (the duodenum, jejunum, and ileum together constitute the small intestine).	Two layers, an outer longitudinal and an inner circular.	Raised up into folds — the plicae circulares which do not disappear on stretching; plicae low; glands of Brunner.	Two layers; thin.	Projects into villi; contains characteristic capillary bed in villi; central lacteal in villi; smooth muscle fibres; glands (crypts) present. Some lymph nodules.	Simple columnar type; 2 kinds of cells: 1. Columnar, with terminal bars and striated border. 2. Goblet, secrete mucus. Glands called crypts of Lieberkühn opening between villi; shorter than glands of stomach mucosa.	Glands of Brunner in submucosa; crypts in mucosa. Crypts have Paneth cells and argentaffin cells; they secrete digestive enzymes.	1. villi 2. two kinds of cells in epithelium 3. goblet cells 4. plicae 5. crypts 6. abundant villi (cf. jejunum and ileum) 7. short leaf-shaped villi 8. glands of Brunner
JEJUNUM	As for duodenum	Raised up into the tallest plicae of small intestine; very vascular.	As for duodenum.	As for duodenum.	As for duodenum.	Crypts only, no glands of Brunner.	1 to 5 – as for duodenum 6. villi less abundant 7. tongue-shaped villi with swollen ends 8. tall plicae

ILEUM (the histological differences between jejunum and ileum are slight).	As for duodenum	Fewer plicae, none in lower region. Peyer's patches extend into submucosa in places.	As for duodenum.	As for duodenum, except for lymph nodules which are aggregated together as Peyer's patches.	As for duodenum.	As for jejunum.	1 to 5 – as for duodenum 6. villi less abundant still 7. finger-shaped villi 8. plicae few or none 9. Peyer's patches
COLON	Two layers, an outer longitudinal and an inner circular. Three bands of fibres occur in longitudinal layer, the taeniae. These are equally spaced apart (120° in cross section) but are shorter than colon. Except for taeniae the muscularis layer is thin.	No plicae; lymph nodules may project into submucosa.	As for duodenum.	Thicker than in small intestine; no villi; numerous tubular glands; large lymph nodules.	Simple columnar; very few goblet cells present.	Simple tubular glands (crypts of Lieberkühn) in lamina propria, regularly arranged in rows; profusion of goblet cells characteristic feature; glands longer than those of stomach or small intestine; glands secrete mucus.	1. no villi 2. few goblet cells in epithelium 3. long tubular glands 4. abundant goblet cells in glands 5. taeniae (in LS they may be cut along their length or not at all) 6. thin muscularis externa 7. large lumen 8. Peyer's patches project into submucosa
APPENDIX	As for duodenum	Lymphatic tissue projects into the submucosa.	Not well developed; may be absent in places.	Contains large amount of lymphatic tissue which may form a continuous circular zone. Eosinophilic leucocytes plentiful.	Simple columnar; few goblet cells present.	Crypts fewer; goblet cells sparsely scattered.	1. ring of lymphatic tissue 2. narrow lumen (may be obliterated) 3. lymphocytes between crypts
RECTUM	No taeniae: layer much thicker than in colon.	A few isolated lymph nodules; small veins in anal canal may dilate and bulge into lumen as haemorrhoids.	Absent in anal canal; lamina propria and submucosa merge here; well-developed in rectum.	Thicker than in colon.	Becomes stratified squamous towards recto-anal junction; thrown into longitudinal folds.	As for colon except for size of glands, which are largest of alimentary canal. Glands absent in junction zone.	1 to 4 – as for colon 5. no taeniae 6. thick muscularis externa 7. longest glands 8. epithelium becomes stratified near recto-anal junction

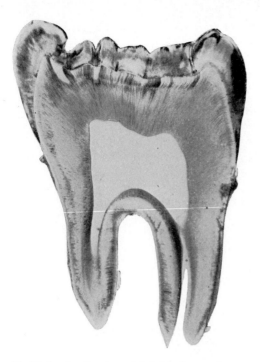

31. **Molar tooth, ground,** L.S. (man), mag. 6x

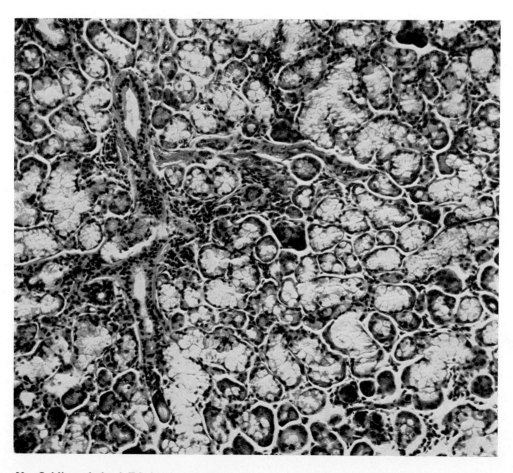

32. **Sublingual gland,** T.S. (man), mag. 150x

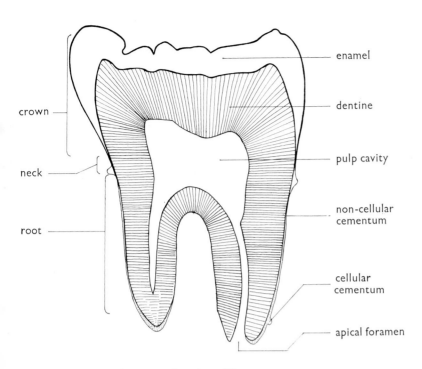

enamel

dentine

pulp cavity

non-cellular cementum

cellular cementum

apical foramen

crown

neck

root

Drawing of specimen 31

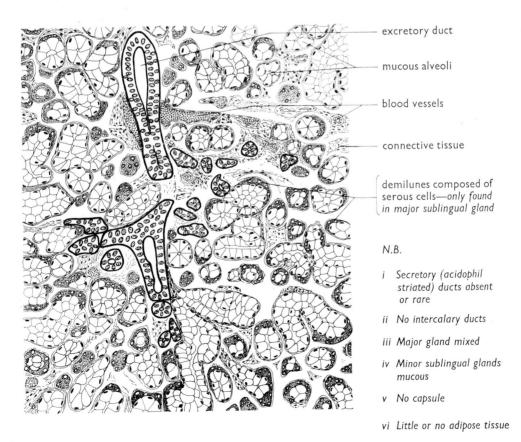

excretory duct

mucous alveoli

blood vessels

connective tissue

demilunes composed of serous cells—*only found in major sublingual gland*

N.B.

i *Secretory (acidophil striated) ducts absent or rare*

ii *No intercalary ducts*

iii *Major gland mixed*

iv *Minor sublingual glands mucous*

v *No capsule*

vi *Little or no adipose tissue*

Drawing of specimen 32

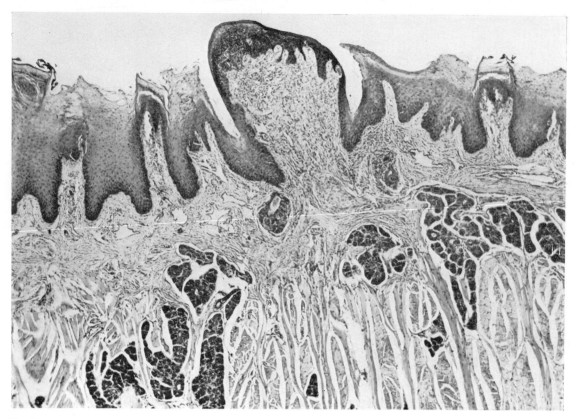

33. **Tongue,** V.S. (man), mag. 38x

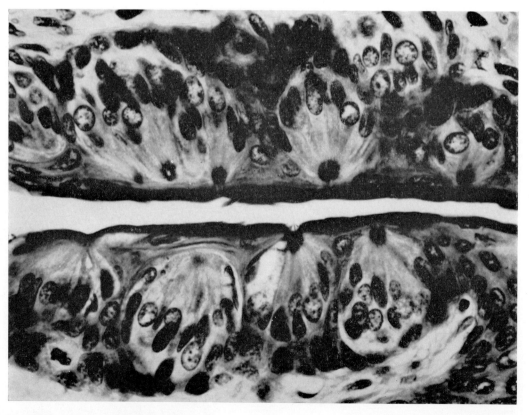

34. **Taste buds,** V.S. (rabbit), mag. 850x

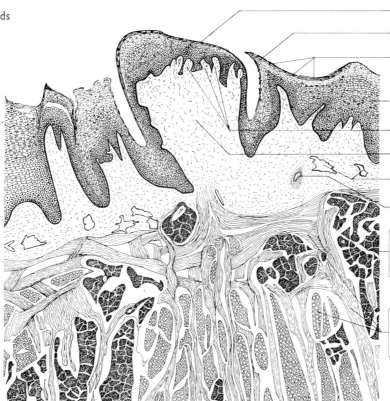

...ribution of Taste Buds

...liform papilla
...aste buds absent

...ngiform papilla
...ew taste buds

...mvallate papilla
...taste buds

...te papillae
...taste buds

...te papilla less
...ounced in man,
...picuous in rabbit)

fungiform papilla

filiform papilla

hard—*but non-keratinised* scales which are shed

stratified squamous epithelium

secondary papillae

primary papilla

blood vessels

duct of lingual gland

lingual gland—*serous type = gland of von Ebner, ducts open into moats of circumvallate papillae*

striated muscle fibres— *the fibres are arranged in vertical, transverse and longitudinal bundles*

N.B. There is no distinct submucosa in the tongue

Drawing of specimen 33

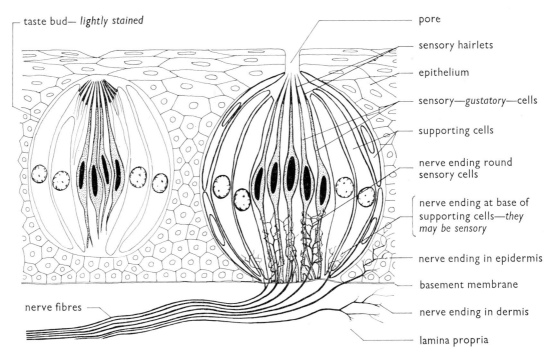

taste bud— *lightly stained*

nerve fibres

pore

sensory hairlets

epithelium

sensory—*gustatory*—cells

supporting cells

nerve ending round sensory cells

nerve ending at base of supporting cells—*they may be sensory*

nerve ending in epidermis

basement membrane

nerve ending in dermis

lamina propria

Drawing of specimen 34

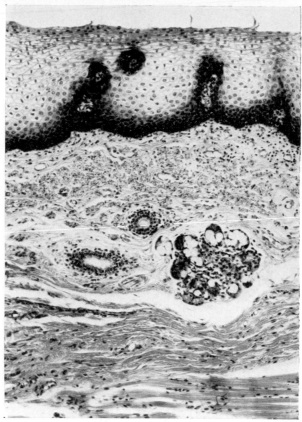

35. **Oesophagus wall,** T.S. (man), mag. 34x

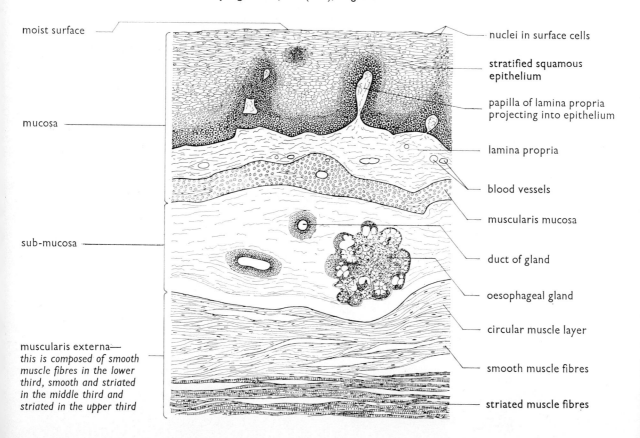

moist surface

mucosa

sub-mucosa

muscularis externa—
*this is composed of smooth
muscle fibres in the lower
third, smooth and striated
in the middle third and
striated in the upper third*

nuclei in surface cells

stratified squamous
epithelium

papilla of lamina propria
projecting into epithelium

lamina propria

blood vessels

muscularis mucosa

duct of gland

oesophageal gland

circular muscle layer

smooth muscle fibres

striated muscle fibres

Drawing of specimen 35

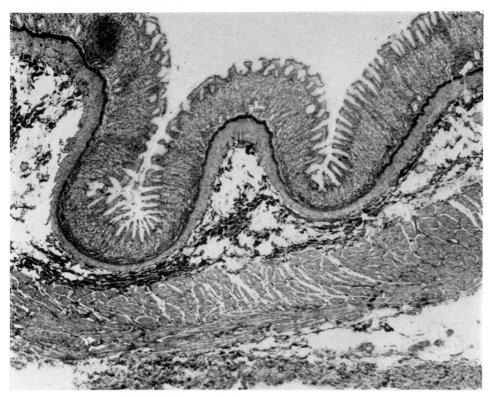

36. Stomach wall, cardiac region, L.S. (man), mag. 42x

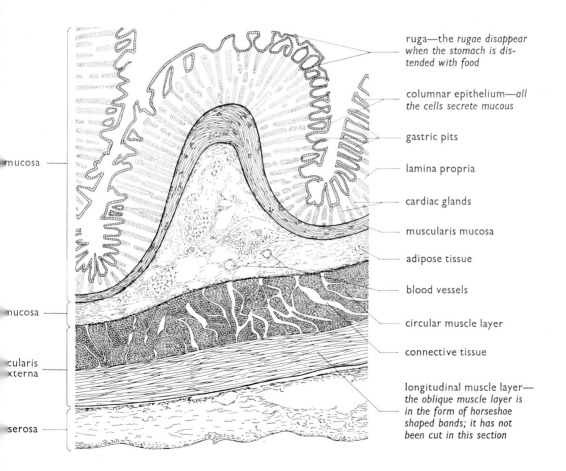

ruga—the *rugae disappear when the stomach is distended with food*

columnar epithelium—*all the cells secrete mucous*

gastric pits

lamina propria

cardiac glands

muscularis mucosa

adipose tissue

blood vessels

circular muscle layer

connective tissue

longitudinal muscle layer—*the oblique muscle layer is in the form of horseshoe shaped bands; it has not been cut in this section*

mucosa

mucosa

cularis xterna

serosa

Drawing of specimen 36

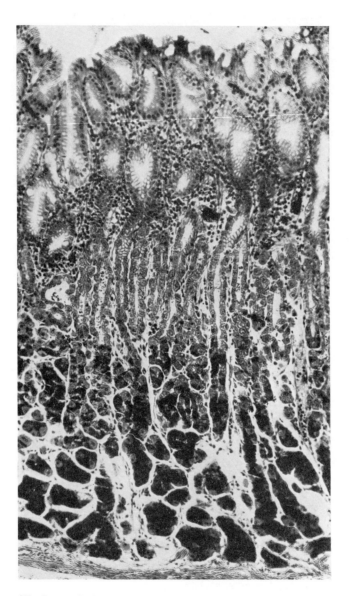

37. **Stomach,** fundic region, mucosa, L.S. (man), mag. 100x

Diagram of a fundic gland

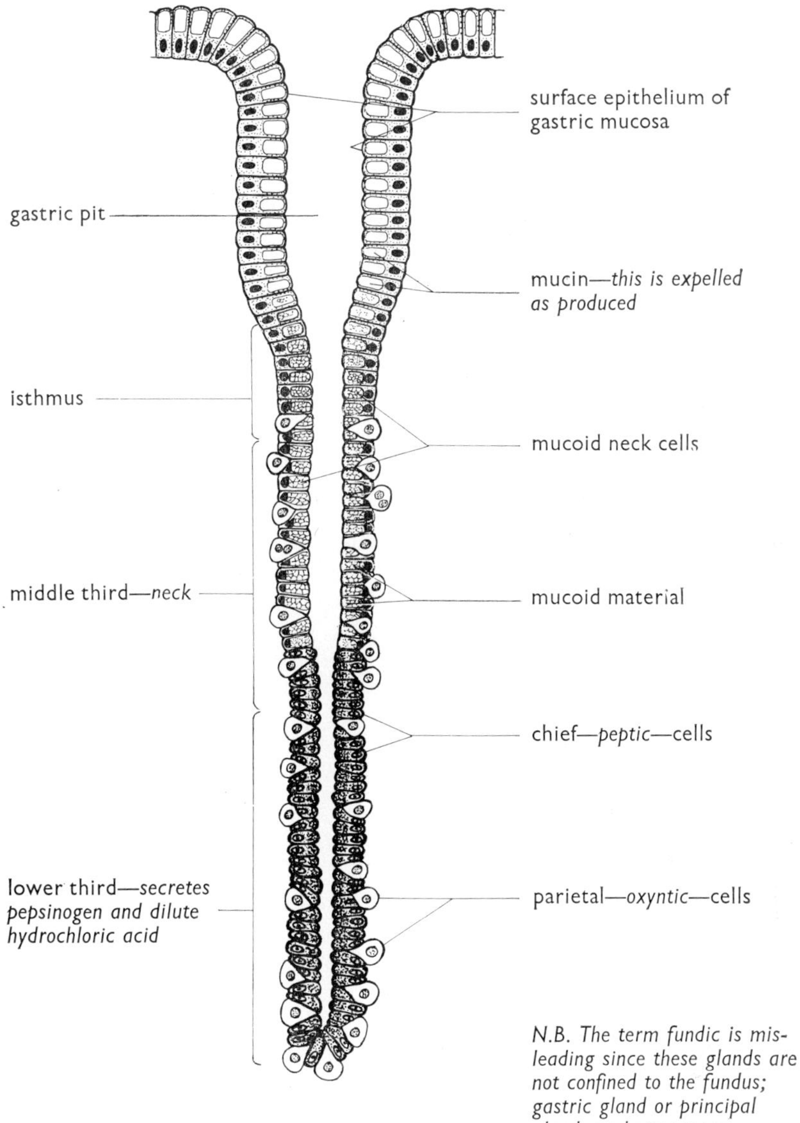

surface epithelium of
gastric mucosa

gastric pit

mucin—*this is expelled
as produced*

isthmus

mucoid neck cells

middle third—*neck*

mucoid material

chief—*peptic*—cells

lower third—*secretes
pepsinogen and dilute
hydrochloric acid*

parietal—*oxyntic*—cells

*N.B. The term fundic is mis-
leading since these glands are
not confined to the fundus;
gastric gland or principal
gland are better terms.*

Drawing of specimen 37

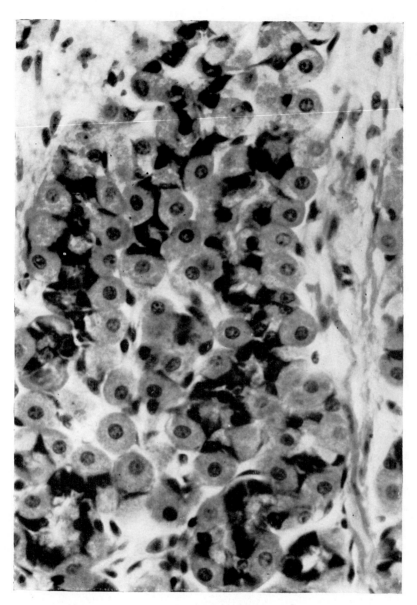

38. **Stomach,** fundic gland detail, L.S. (man), mag. 850x

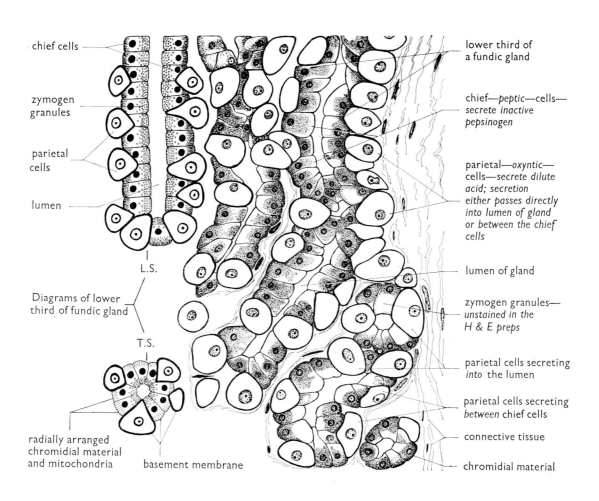

chief cells

zymogen
granules

parietal
cells

lumen

L.S.

Diagrams of lower
third of fundic gland

T.S.

radially arranged
chromidial material
and mitochondria

basement membrane

lower third of
a fundic gland

chief—*peptic*—cells—
*secrete inactive
pepsinogen*

parietal—*oxyntic*—
cells—*secrete dilute
acid; secretion
either passes directly
into lumen of gland
or between the chief
cells*

lumen of gland

zymogen granules—
*unstained in the
H & E preps*

parietal cells secreting
into the lumen

parietal cells secreting
between chief cells

connective tissue

chromidial material

Drawing of specimen 38

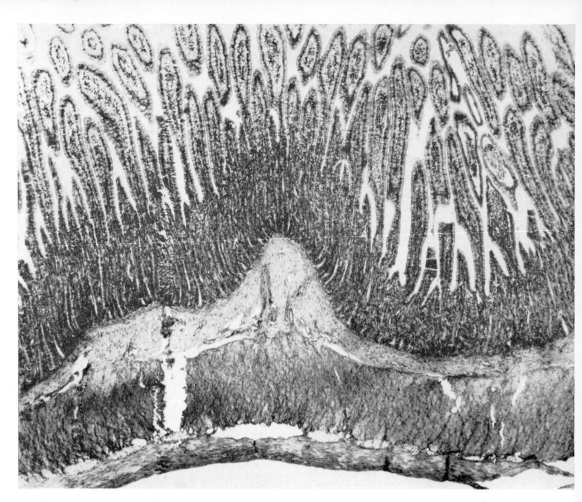

39. **Ileum,** L.S. (man), mag. 32x

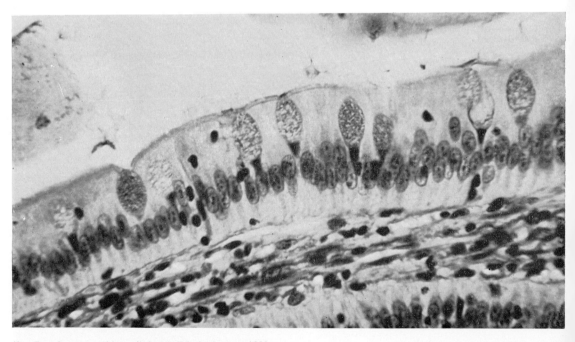

40. **Duodenum,** goblet cell detail, T.S. (cat), mag. 1000x

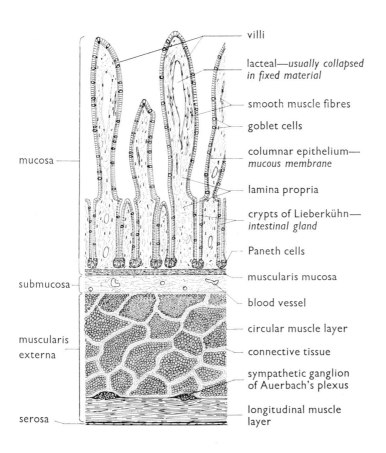

villi

lacteal—*usually collapsed in fixed material*

smooth muscle fibres

goblet cells

columnar epithelium—*mucous membrane*

lamina propria

crypts of Lieberkühn—*intestinal gland*

Paneth cells

muscularis mucosa

blood vessel

circular muscle layer

connective tissue

sympathetic ganglion of Auerbach's plexus

longitudinal muscle layer

mucosa

submucosa

muscularis externa

serosa

Drawing of specimen 39

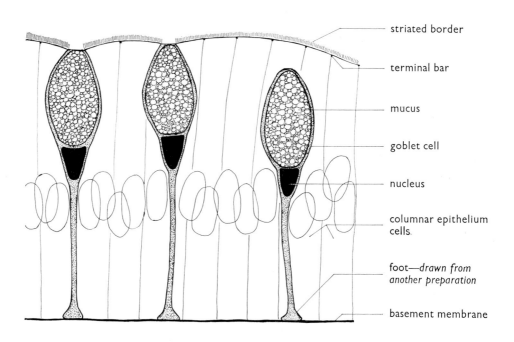

striated border

terminal bar

mucus

goblet cell

nucleus

columnar epithelium cells.

foot—*drawn from another preparation*

basement membrane

Drawing of specimen 40

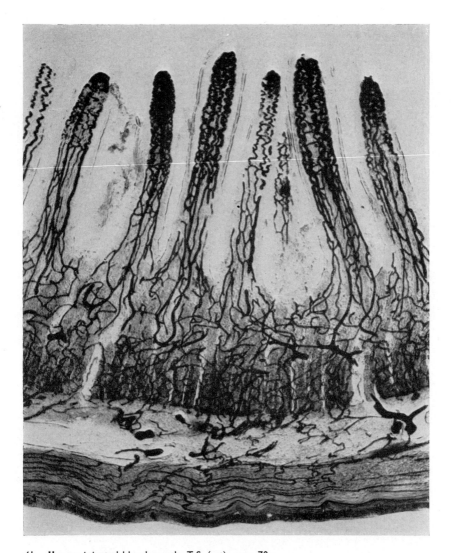

41. **Ileum,** injected blood vessels, T.S. (cat), mag. 70x

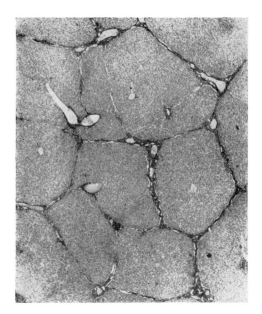

42. **Liver,** to show lobules, T.S. (pig), mag. 30x

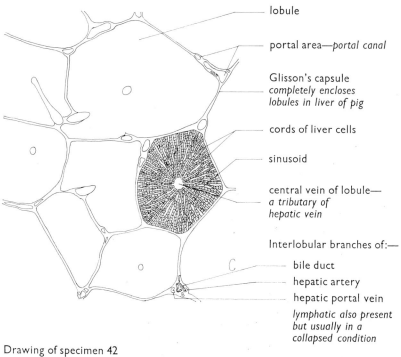

lobule

portal area—*portal canal*

Glisson's capsule
*completely encloses
lobules in liver of pig*

cords of liver cells

sinusoid

central vein of lobule—
*a tributary of
hepatic vein*

Interlobular branches of:—

bile duct
hepatic artery
hepatic portal vein
*lymphatic also present
but usually in a
collapsed condition*

Drawing of specimen 42

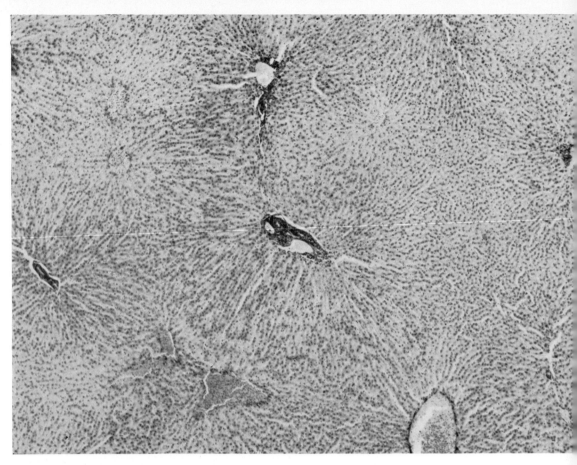

43. **Liver,** T.S. (man), mag. 60x

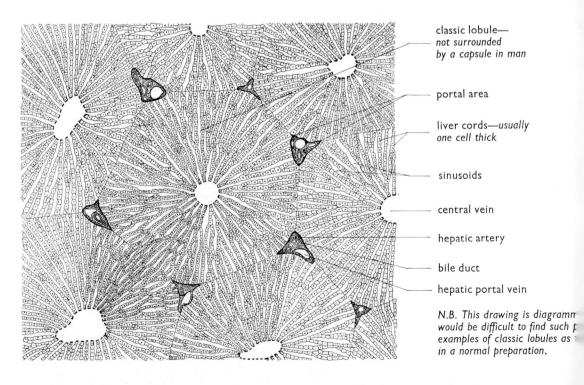

classic lobule—
*not surrounded
by a capsule in man*

portal area

liver cords—*usually
one cell thick*

sinusoids

central vein

hepatic artery

bile duct

hepatic portal vein

*N.B. This drawing is diagramm
would be difficult to find such p
examples of classic lobules as
in a normal preparation.*

Drawing of specimen 43

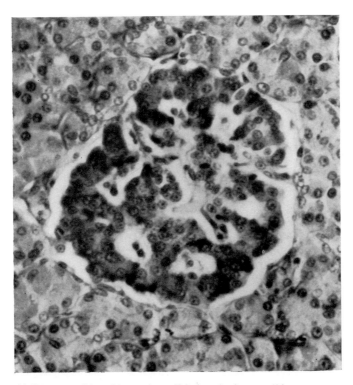

44 **Pancreas,** Islet of Langerhans, T.S. (monkey), mag. 420x

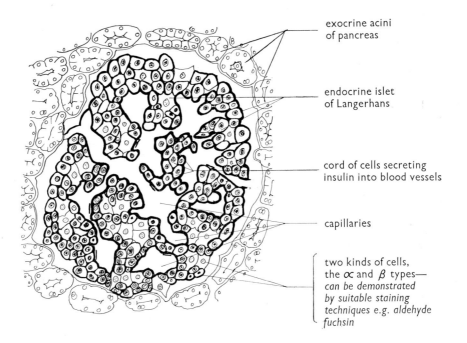

exocrine acini
of pancreas

endocrine islet
of Langerhans

cord of cells secreting
insulin into blood vessels

capillaries

two kinds of cells,
the α and β types—
*can be demonstrated
by suitable staining
techniques e.g. aldehyde
fuchsin*

Drawing of specimen 44

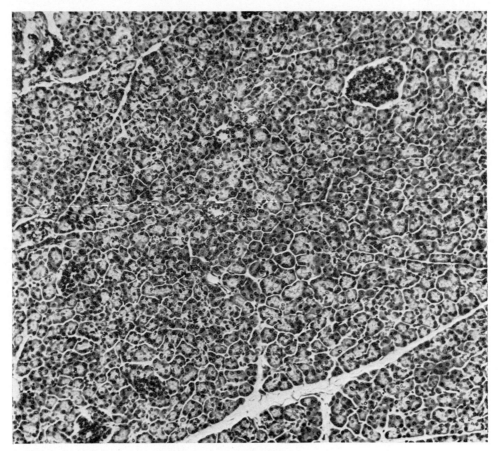

45. **Pancreas,** T. S. (monkey), mag. 65x

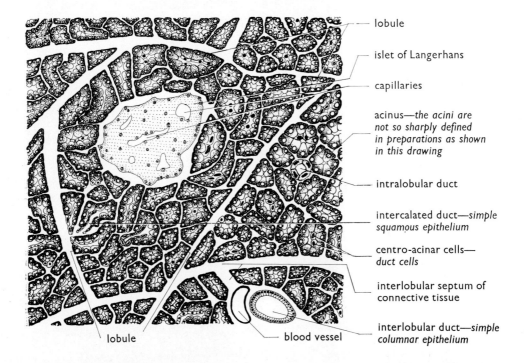

lobule

islet of Langerhans

capillaries

acinus—*the acini are
not so sharply defined
in preparations as shown
in this drawing*

intralobular duct

intercalated duct—*simple
squamous epithelium*

centro-acinar cells—
duct cells

interlobular septum of
connective tissue

interlobular duct—*simple
columnar epithelium*

lobule

blood vessel

Drawing of specimen 45

THE UROGENITAL SYSTEM

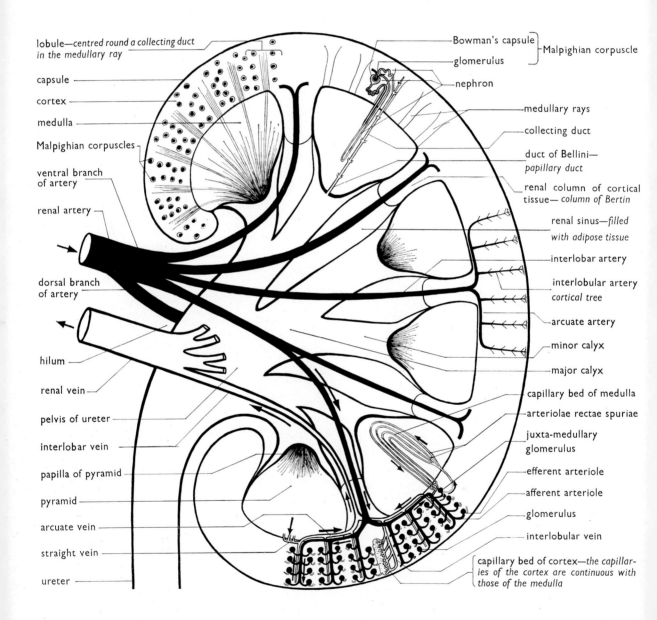

lobule—*centred round a collecting duct in the medullary ray*

capsule

cortex

medulla

Malpighian corpuscles

ventral branch of artery

renal artery

dorsal branch of artery

hilum

renal vein

pelvis of ureter

interlobar vein

papilla of pyramid

pyramid

arcuate vein

straight vein

ureter

Bowman's capsule

glomerulus

Malpighian corpuscle

nephron

medullary rays

collecting duct

duct of Bellini— *papillary duct*

renal column of cortical tissue— *column of Bertin*

renal sinus—*filled with adipose tissue*

interlobar artery

interlobular artery *cortical tree*

arcuate artery

minor calyx

major calyx

capillary bed of medulla

arteriolae rectae spuriae

juxta-medullary glomerulus

efferent arteriole

afferent arteriole

glomerulus

interlobular vein

capillary bed of cortex—*the capillaries of the cortex are continuous with those of the medulla*

DIAGRAM TO SHOW THE STRUCTURE AND BLOOD SUPPLY OF THE KIDNEY OF MAN

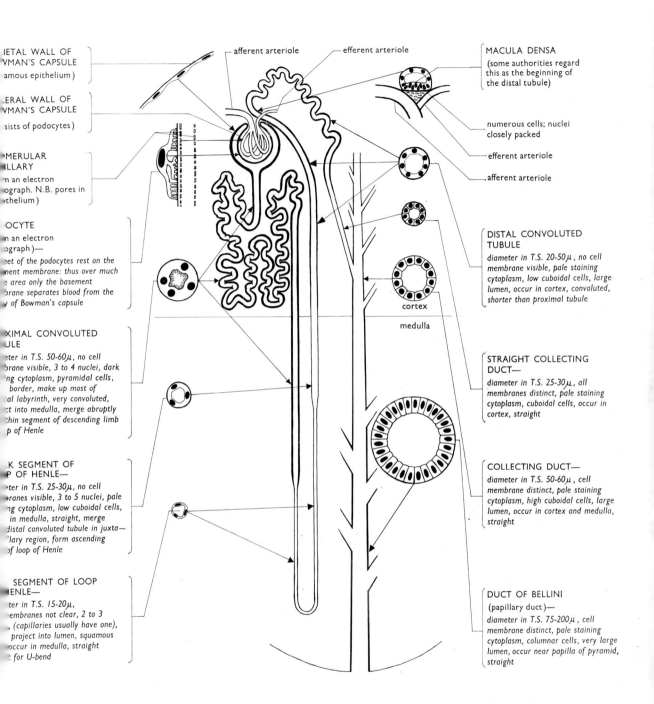

...IETAL WALL OF
...WMAN'S CAPSULE
(...amous epithelium)

...ERAL WALL OF
...WMAN'S CAPSULE
(...sists of podocytes)

...MERULAR
...LLARY
(...m an electron
...ograph. N.B. pores in
...thelium)

...OCYTE
(...m an electron
...ograph)—
...eet of the podocytes rest on the
...ment membrane: thus over much
...e area only the basement
...brane separates blood from the
...y of Bowman's capsule

...XIMAL CONVOLUTED
...ULE
...eter in T.S. 50-60μ, no cell
...brane visible, 3 to 4 nuclei, dark
...ng cytoplasm, pyramidal cells,
...border, make up most of
...al labyrinth, very convoluted,
...ct into medulla, merge abruptly
...thin segment of descending limb
...p of Henle

...K SEGMENT OF
...P OF HENLE—
...ter in T.S. 25-30μ, no cell
...ranes visible, 3 to 5 nuclei, pale
...ng cytoplasm, low cuboidal cells,
...in medulla, straight, merge
...distal convoluted tubule in juxta—
...lary region, form ascending
...of loop of Henle

...SEGMENT OF LOOP
...ENLE—
...ter in T.S. 15-20μ,
...embranes not clear, 2 to 3
...(capillaries usually have one),
...project into lumen, squamous
...occur in medulla, straight
...for U-bend

afferent arteriole

efferent arteriole

MACULA DENSA
(some authorities regard
this as the beginning of
the distal tubule)

numerous cells; nuclei
closely packed

efferent arteriole

afferent arteriole

DISTAL CONVOLUTED
TUBULE
diameter in T.S. 20-50μ, no cell
membrane visible, pale staining
cytoplasm, low cuboidal cells, large
lumen, occur in cortex, convoluted,
shorter than proximal tubule

cortex

medulla

STRAIGHT COLLECTING
DUCT—
diameter in T.S. 25-30μ, all
membranes distinct, pale staining
cytoplasm, cuboidal cells, occur in
cortex, straight

COLLECTING DUCT—
diameter in T.S. 50-60μ, cell
membrane distinct, pale staining
cytoplasm, high cuboidal cells, large
lumen, occur in cortex and medulla,
straight

DUCT OF BELLINI
(papillary duct)—
diameter in T.S. 75-200μ, cell
membrane distinct, pale staining
cytoplasm, columnar cells, very large
lumen, occur near papilla of pyramid,
straight

DIAGRAM OF A NEPHRON

A nephron consists of Bowman's
capsule, glomerulus, proximal
convoluted tubule, loop of Henle
and distal convoluted tubule.

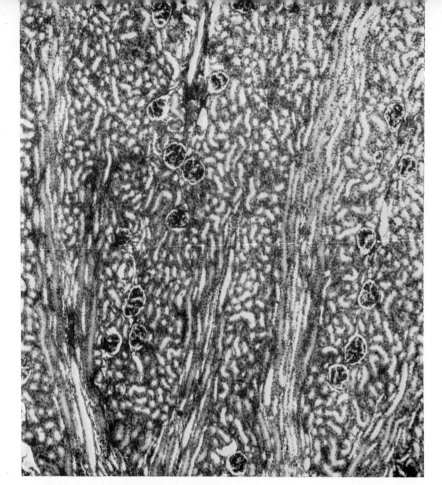

46. **Kidney,** cortex, L.S. (monkey), mag.40x

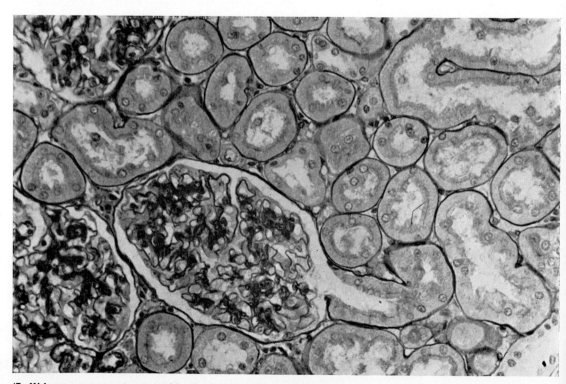

47. **Kidney,** cortex, section stained by the P.A.S. technique (rat), mag. 560x

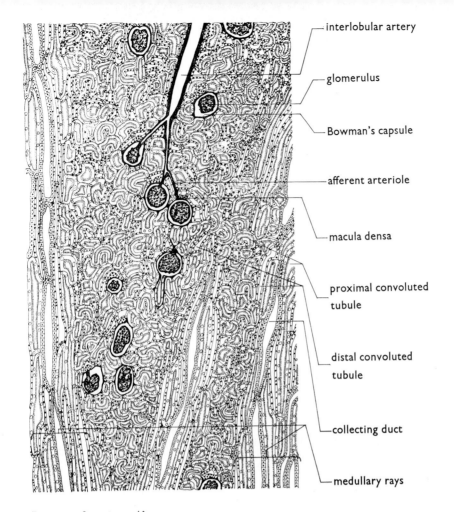

- interlobular artery
- glomerulus
- Bowman's capsule
- afferent arteriole
- macula densa
- proximal convoluted tubule
- distal convoluted tubule
- collecting duct
- medullary rays

Drawing of specimen 46

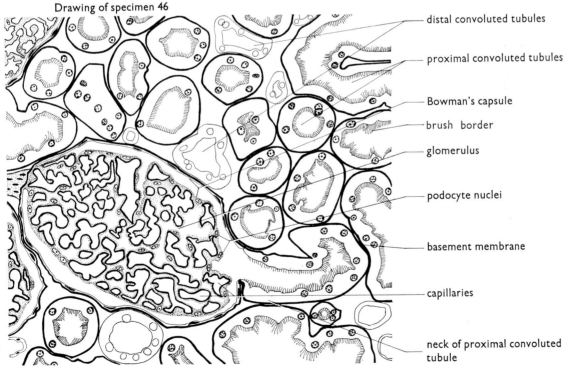

- distal convoluted tubules
- proximal convoluted tubules
- Bowman's capsule
- brush border
- glomerulus
- podocyte nuclei
- basement membrane
- capillaries
- neck of proximal convoluted tubule

Drawing of specimen 47

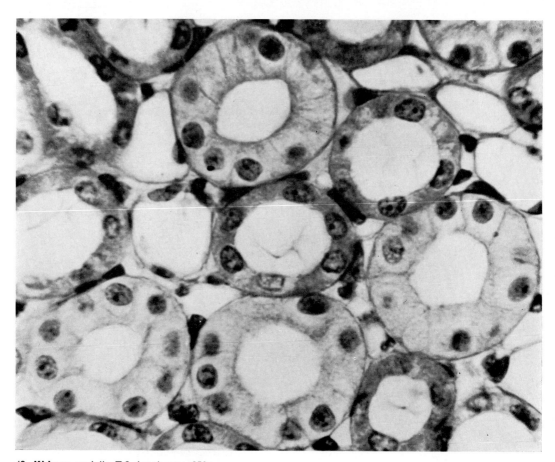

48. **Kidney,** medulla, T.S. (man), mag. 850x

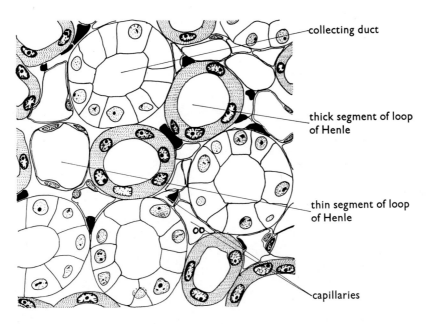

collecting duct

thick segment of loop of Henle

thin segment of loop of Henle

capillaries

Drawing of specimen 48

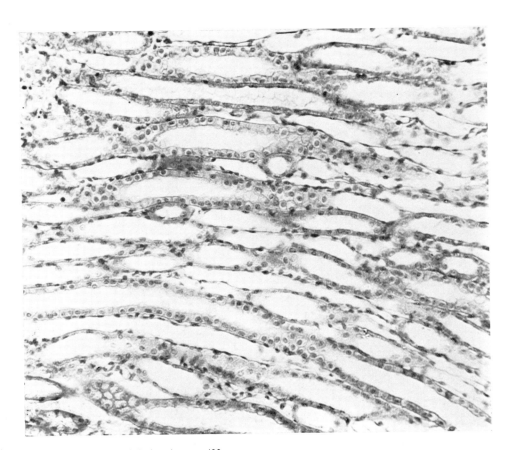

49. **Kidney,** medulla, L.S. (man), mag. 400x

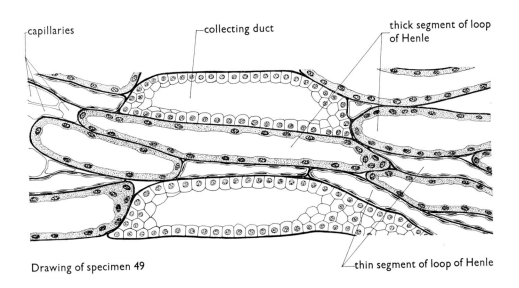

capillaries

collecting duct

thick segment of loop of Henle

Drawing of specimen 49

thin segment of loop of Henle

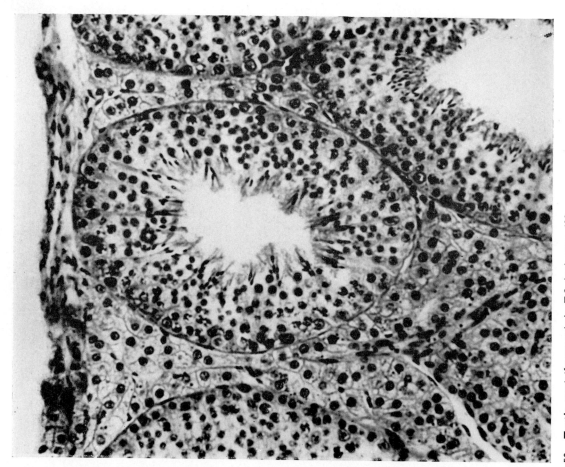

50. **Testis**, seminiferous tubule, T.S. (cat), mag. 400x

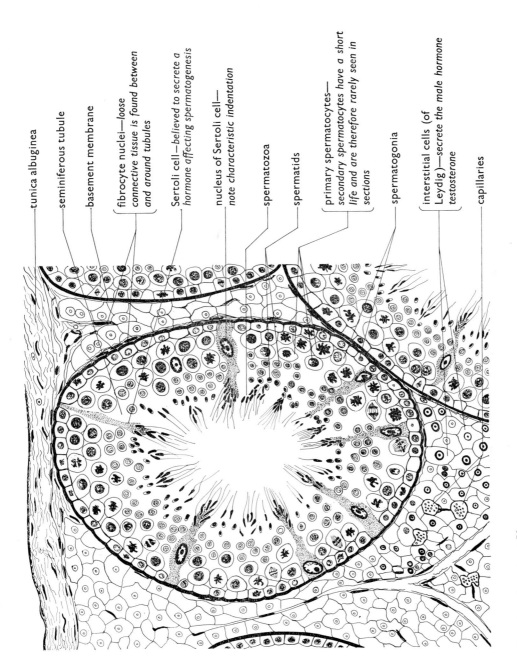

tunica albuginea

seminiferous tubule

basement membrane

fibrocyte nuclei—loose connective tissue is found between and around tubules

Sertoli cell—believed to secrete a hormone affecting spermatogenesis

nucleus of Sertoli cell—note characteristic indentation

spermatozoa

spermatids

primary spermatocytes—secondary spermatocytes have a short life and are therefore rarely seen in sections

spermatogonia

interstitial cells (of Leydig)—secrete the male hormone testosterone

capillaries

Drawing of specimen 50

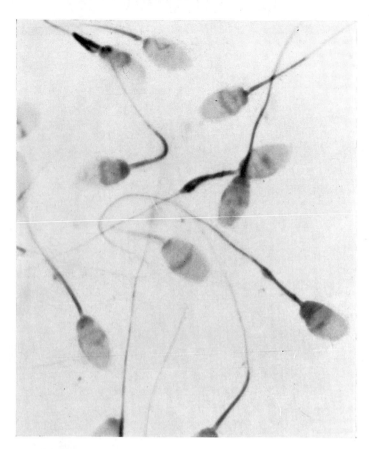

51. **Spermatozoa,** E. (guinea pig), mag. 1900x

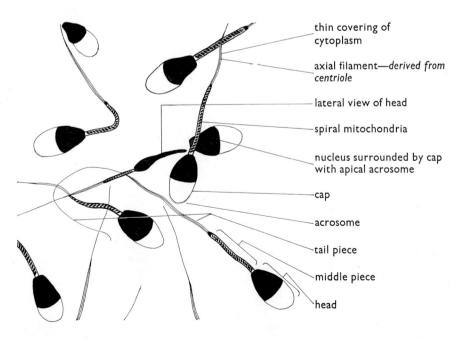

thin covering of cytoplasm

axial filament—*derived from centriole*

lateral view of head

spiral mitochondria

nucleus surrounded by cap with apical acrosome

cap

acrosome

tail piece

middle piece

head

Drawing of specimen 51

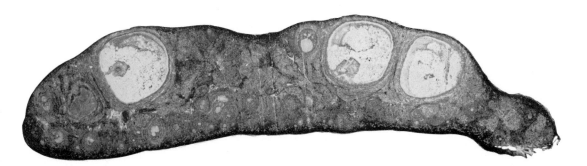

52. **Ovary,** L.S. (rabbit), mag. 12x

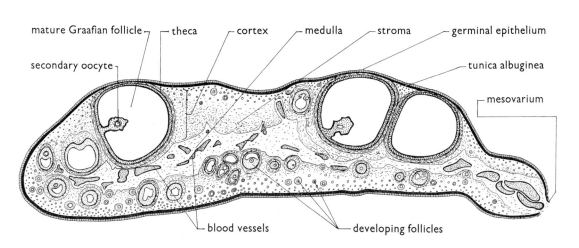

mature Graafian follicle — — theca — cortex — medulla — stroma — germinal epithelium

secondary oocyte — — tunica albuginea

— mesovarium

— blood vessels — developing follicles

Drawing of specimen 52

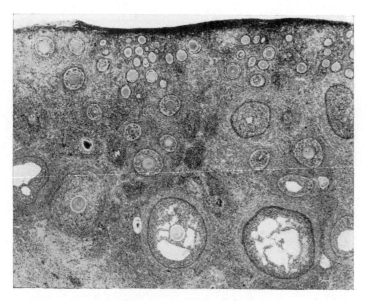

53. **Ovary,** developing follicle, L.S. (rabbit), mag. 170x

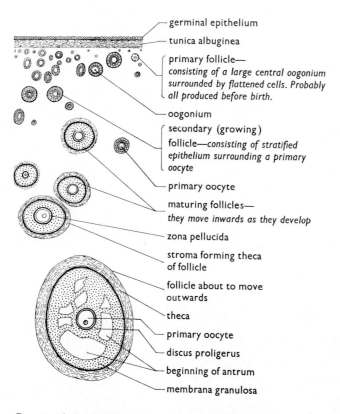

germinal epithelium

tunica albuginea

primary follicle—
consisting of a large central oogonium surrounded by flattened cells. Probably all produced before birth.

oogonium

secondary (growing)
follicle—*consisting of stratified epithelium surrounding a primary oocyte*

primary oocyte

maturing follicles—
they move inwards as they develop

zona pellucida

stroma forming theca of follicle

follicle about to move outwards

theca

primary oocyte

discus proligerus

beginning of antrum

membrana granulosa

Drawing of specimen 53

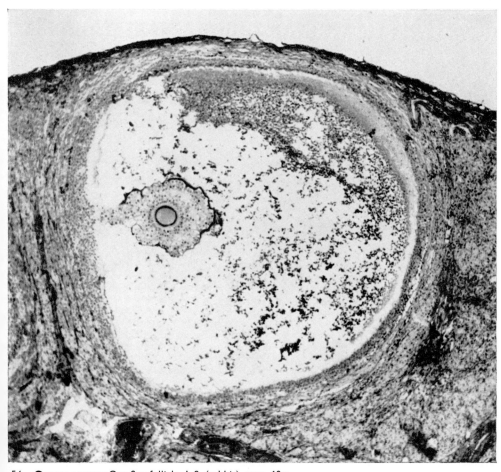

54. Ovary, matrue Graafian follicle, L.S. (rabbit), mag. 60x

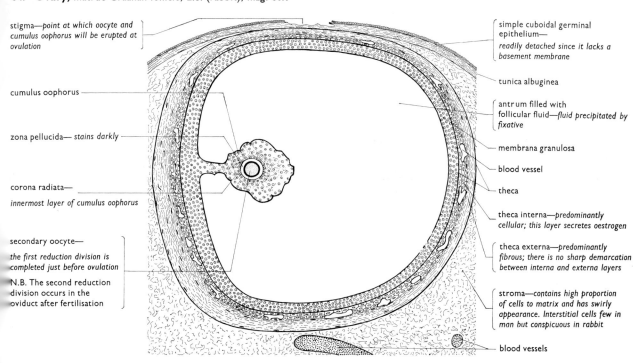

stigma—*point at which oocyte and cumulus oophorus will be erupted at ovulation*

cumulus oophorus

zona pellucida— *stains darkly*

corona radiata—

innermost layer of cumulus oophorus

secondary oocyte—

the first reduction division is completed just before ovulation

N.B. The second reduction division occurs in the oviduct after fertilisation

simple cuboidal germinal epithelium—

readily detached since it lacks a basement membrane

tunica albuginea

antrum filled with follicular fluid—*fluid precipitated by fixative*

membrana granulosa

blood vessel

theca

theca interna—*predominantly cellular; this layer secretes oestrogen*

theca externa—*predominantly fibrous; there is no sharp demarcation between interna and externa layers*

stroma—*contains high proportion of cells to matrix and has swirly appearance. Interstitial cells few in man but conspicuous in rabbit*

blood vessels

Drawing of specimen 54

88

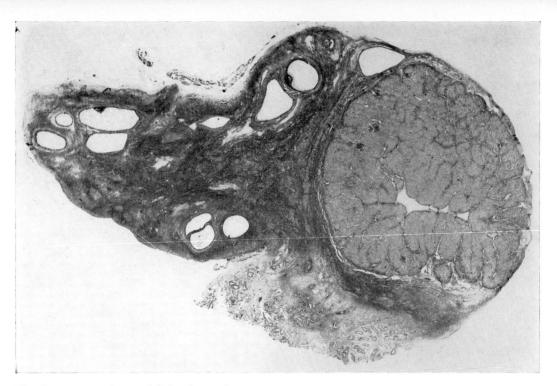

55. **Ovary,** corpus luteum, L.S. (man), mag. 3x

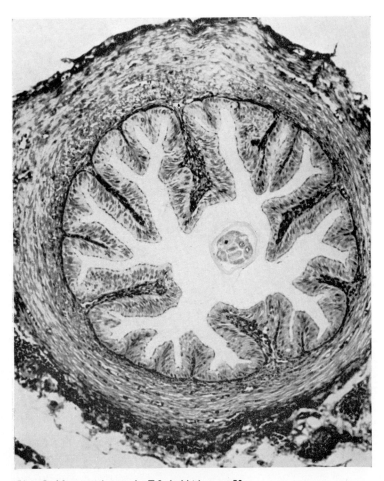

56. **Oviduct,** with morula, T.S. (rabbit), mag. 50x

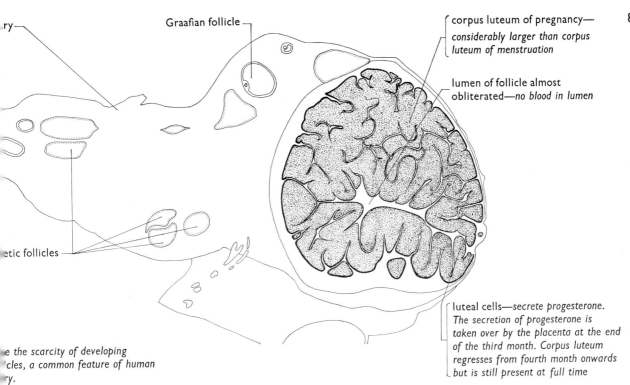

Graafian follicle

ry —

corpus luteum of pregnancy—*considerably larger than corpus luteum of menstruation*

lumen of follicle almost obliterated—*no blood in lumen*

etic follicles

luteal cells—*secrete progesterone. The secretion of progesterone is taken over by the placenta at the end of the third month. Corpus luteum regresses from fourth month onwards but is still present at full time*

e the scarcity of developing
cles, a common feature of human
ry.

wing of specimen 55

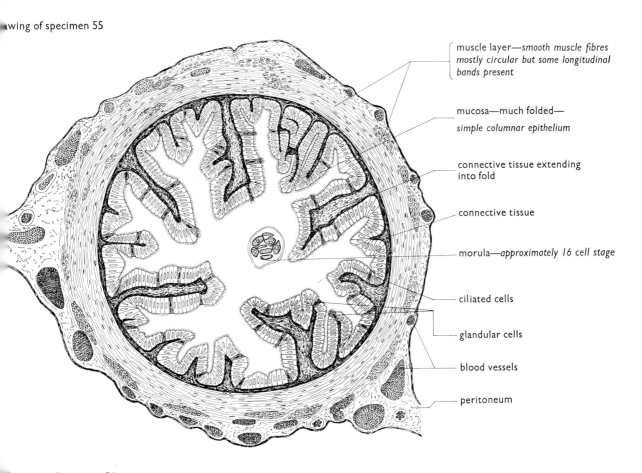

muscle layer—*smooth muscle fibres mostly circular but some longitudinal bands present*

mucosa—much folded—
simple columnar epithelium

connective tissue extending into fold

connective tissue

morula—*approximately 16 cell stage*

ciliated cells

glandular cells

blood vessels

peritoneum

Drawing of specimen 56

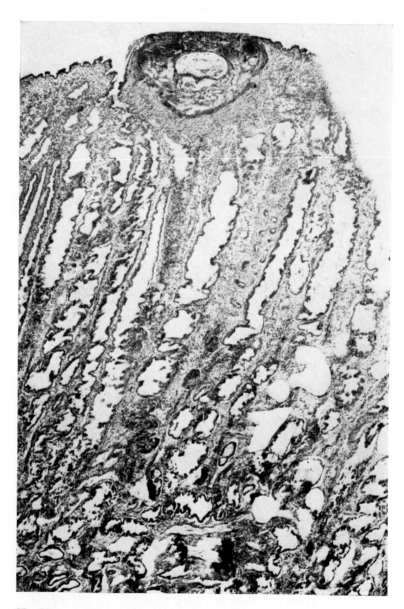

57. **Uterus,** pregnant (man). A previllous human ovum, aged nine to ten days
(the Davies-Harding ovum), mag. 25x (*Preparation and photograph by John Kugler*)

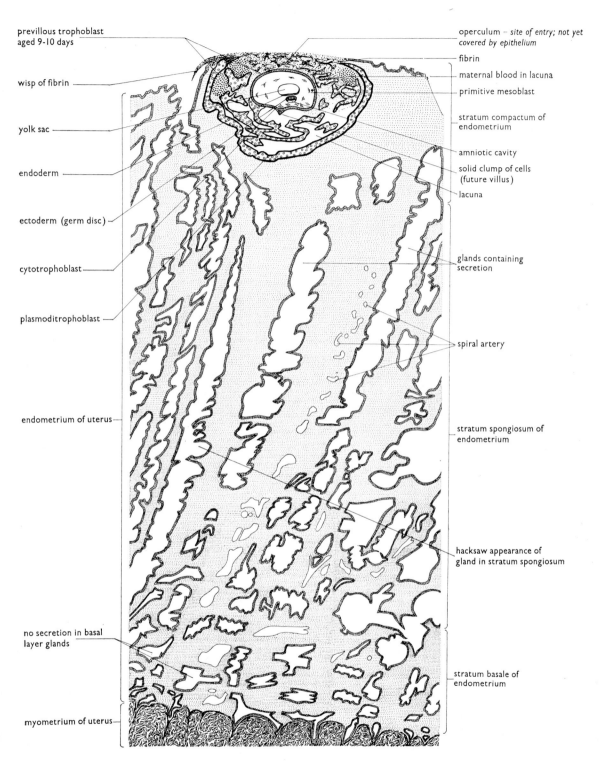

previllous trophoblast
aged 9-10 days

operculum = *site of entry; not yet covered by epithelium*

fibrin

maternal blood in lacuna

wisp of fibrin

primitive mesoblast

stratum compactum of endometrium

yolk sac

endoderm

amniotic cavity

solid clump of cells
(future villus)

ectoderm (germ disc)

lacuna

cytotrophoblast

glands containing
secretion

plasmoditrophoblast

spiral artery

endometrium of uterus

stratum spongiosum of
endometrium

hacksaw appearance of
gland in stratum spongiosum

no secretion in basal
layer glands

stratum basale of
endometrium

myometrium of uterus

Drawing of specimen 57

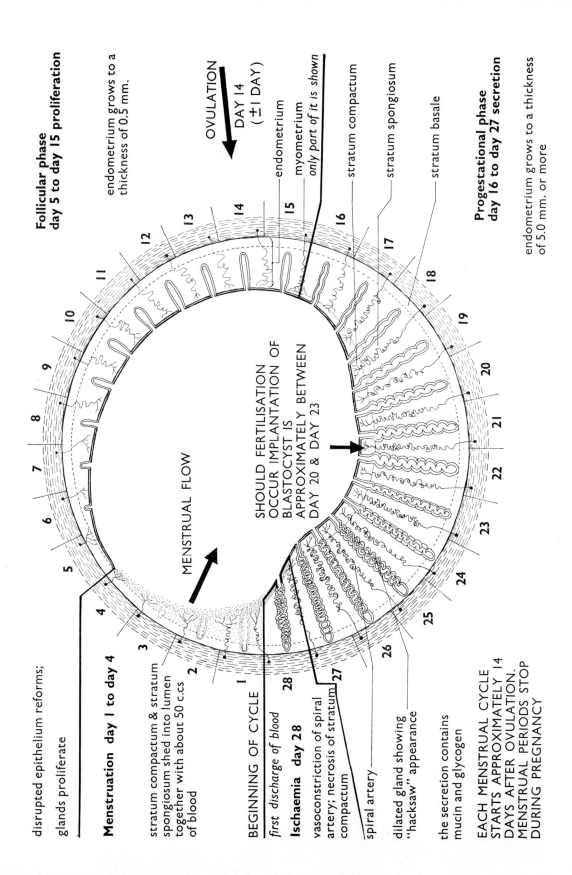

DIAGRAM OF THE CHANGES IN THE ENDOMETRIUM DURING A 28 DAY MENSTRUAL CYCLE

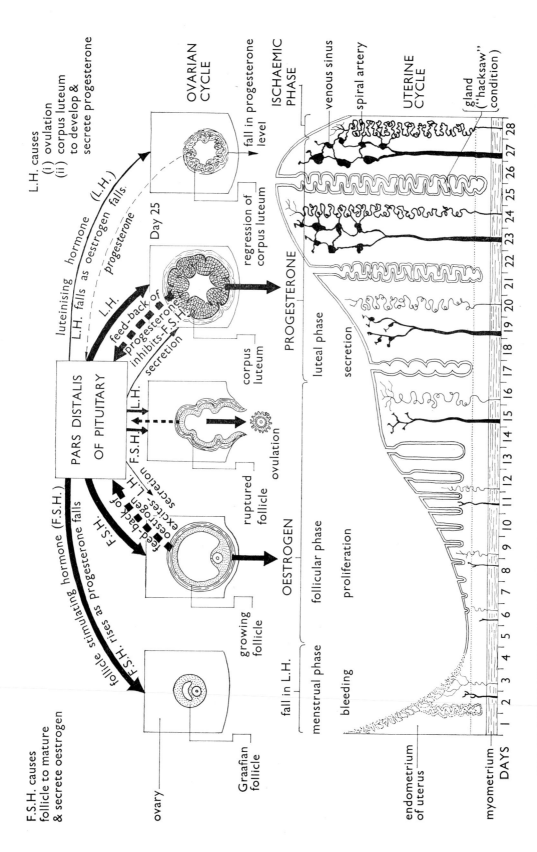

DIAGRAM ILLUSTRATING THE INTEGRATION OF THE OVARIAN AND UTERINE CYCLES BY HORMONES

THE SKIN

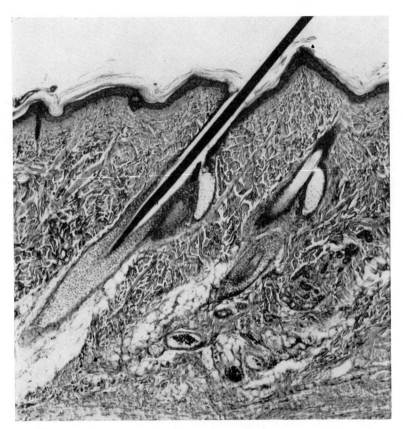

58. **Skin,** gross, hairy, V.S. (baboon), mag. 50x

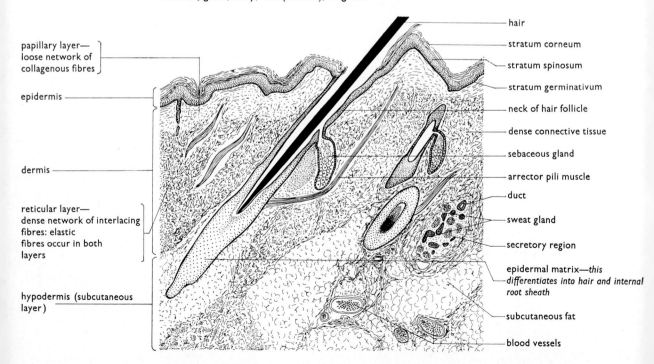

papillary layer—loose network of collagenous fibres

epidermis

dermis

reticular layer—dense network of interlacing fibres: elastic fibres occur in both layers

hypodermis (subcutaneous layer)

hair

stratum corneum

stratum spinosum

stratum germinativum

neck of hair follicle

dense connective tissue

sebaceous gland

arrector pili muscle

duct

sweat gland

secretory region

epidermal matrix—*this differentiates into hair and internal root sheath*

subcutaneous fat

blood vessels

Drawing of specimen 58

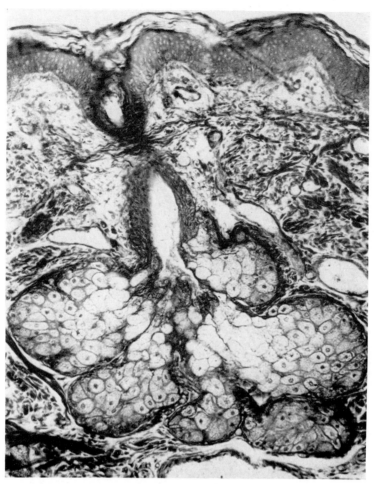

59. **Skin,** hairy, sebaceous gland detail, V.S. (baboon), mag. 10x

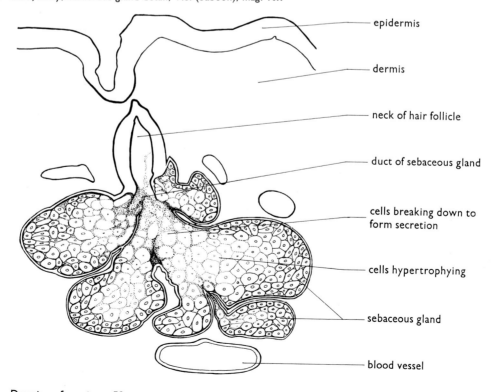

epidermis

dermis

neck of hair follicle

duct of sebaceous gland

cells breaking down to form secretion

cells hypertrophying

sebaceous gland

blood vessel

Drawing of specimen 59

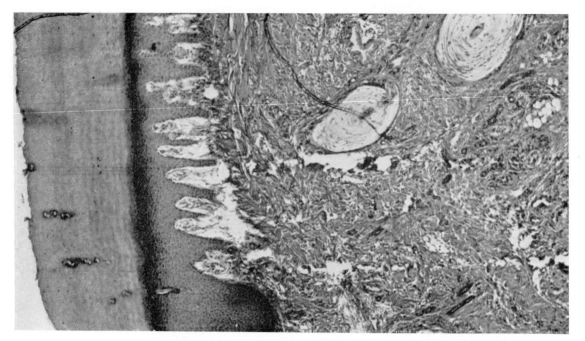

61. **Skin,** non-hairy, finger pad, V.S. (baboon), mag. 70x

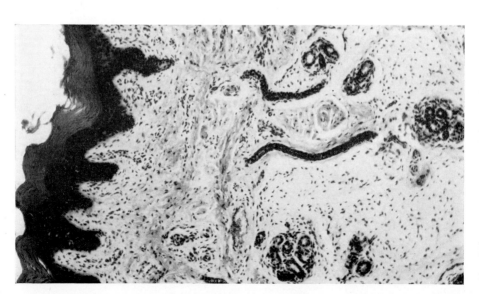

60. **Skin,** non-hairy, sole of foot, for sweat gland detail, V.S. (man), mag. 135x

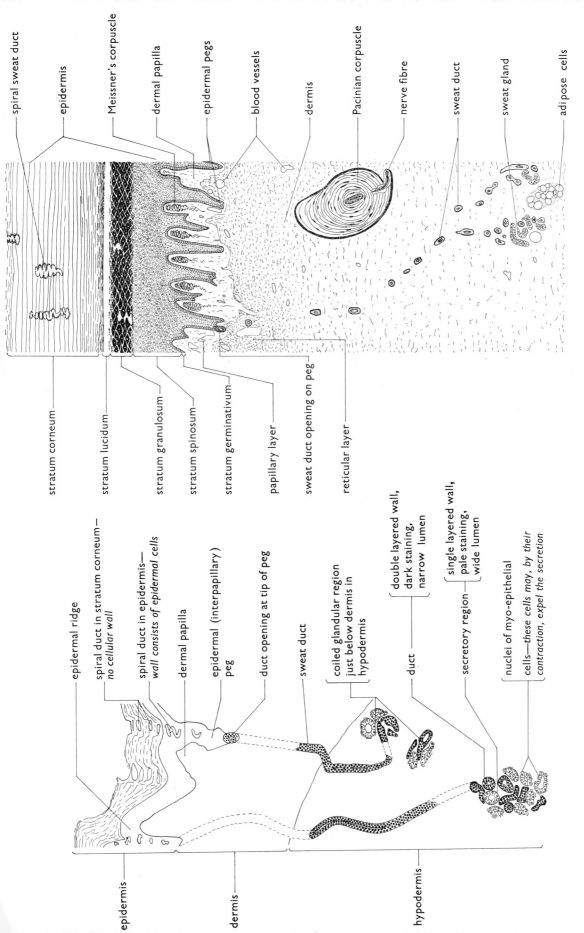

Drawing of specimen 61

Drawing of specimen 60

THE RESPIRATORY SYSTEM

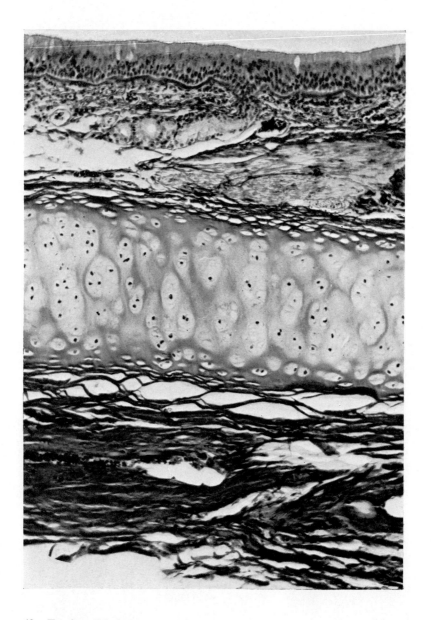

62. **Trachea**, T.S. (man), mag. 170x

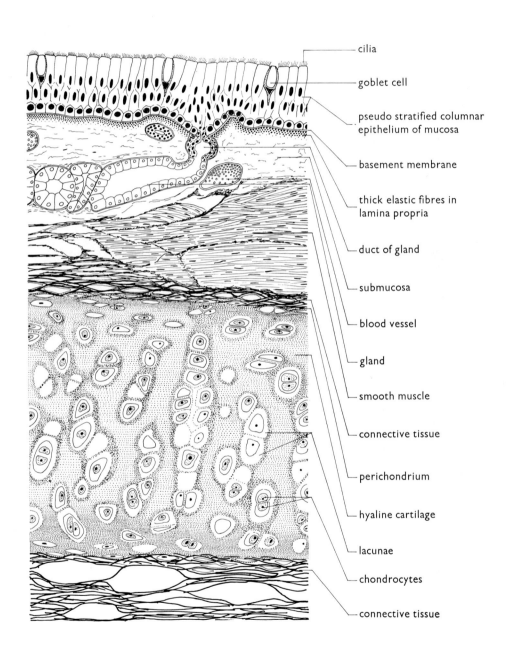

cilia

goblet cell

pseudo stratified columnar
epithelium of mucosa

basement membrane

thick elastic fibres in
lamina propria

duct of gland

submucosa

blood vessel

gland

smooth muscle

connective tissue

perichondrium

hyaline cartilage

lacunae

chondrocytes

connective tissue

Drawing of specimen 62

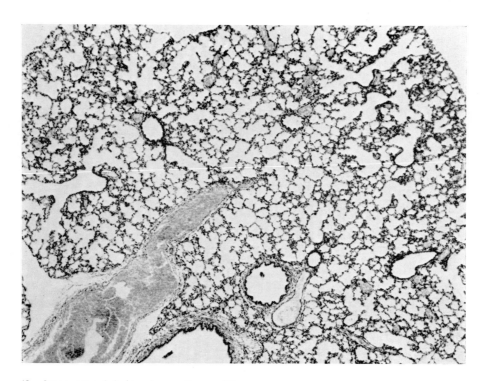

63. **Lung,** gross, L.S. (new-born rat), mag. 22x

	Large bronchus	Small bronchus	Bronchiole	Terminal bronchiole	Respiratory bronchiole	Alveolar duct
Epithelium	pseudo-stratified, ciliated, columnar	pseudo-stratified, ciliated, columnar	pseudo-stratified, ciliated, columnar	simple ciliated columnar	simple cuboidal	simple cuboidal
Goblet cells	present	a few present	very scattered	absent	absent	absent
Cartilage	present	a little present	absent	absent	absent	absent
Glands	present	a few present	absent	absent	absent	absent
Smooth muscle	two sets—a right and a left— spiral		present	present	present	a few fibres present
Alveoli	absent	absent	absent	absent	present	prolific

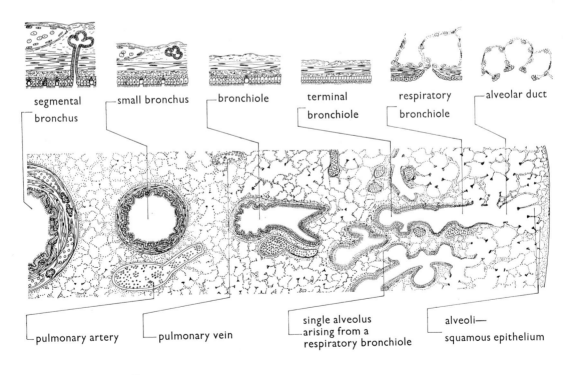

segmental bronchus · small bronchus · bronchiole · terminal bronchiole · respiratory bronchiole · alveolar duct

pulmonary artery · pulmonary vein · single alveolus arising from a respiratory bronchiole · alveoli— squamous epithelium

Drawing of specimen 63

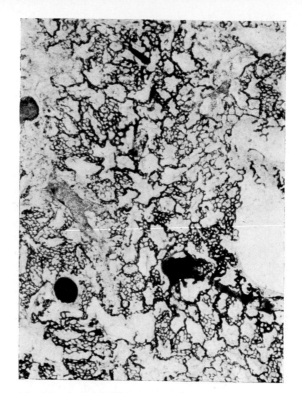

64. **Lung,** injected, T.S. (rat), mag. 100x

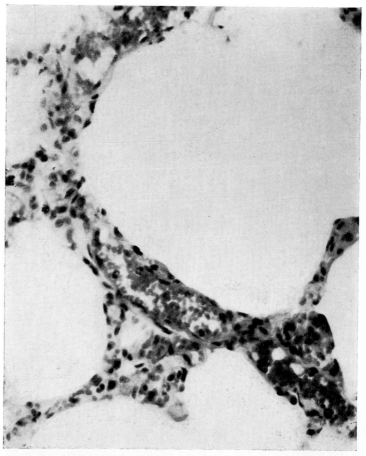

65. **Lung,** high power detail of alveolar wall, T.S. (man), mag. 950x

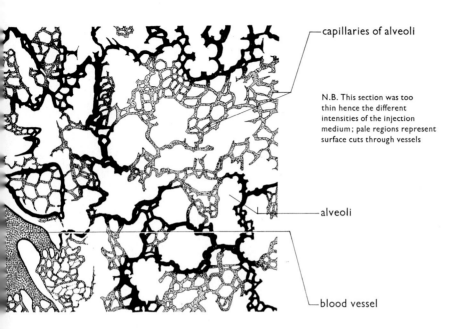

capillaries of alveoli

N.B. This section was too
thin hence the different
intensities of the injection
medium; pale regions represent
surface cuts through vessels

alveoli

blood vessel

Drawing of specimen 64

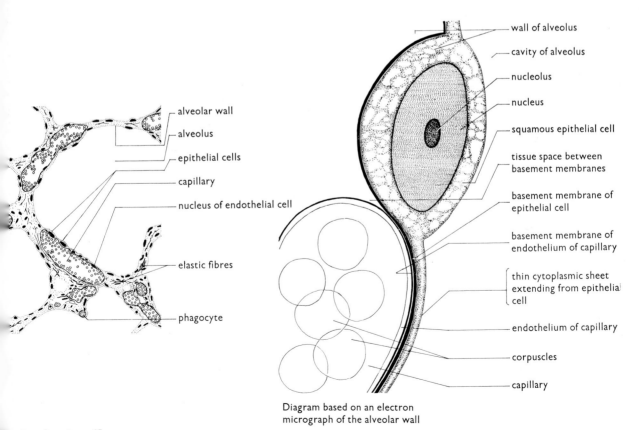

alveolar wall

alveolus

epithelial cells

capillary

nucleus of endothelial cell

elastic fibres

phagocyte

wall of alveolus

cavity of alveolus

nucleolus

nucleus

squamous epithelial cell

tissue space between
basement membranes

basement membrane of
epithelial cell

basement membrane of
endothelium of capillary

thin cytoplasmic sheet
extending from epithelial
cell

endothelium of capillary

corpuscles

capillary

Diagram based on an electron
micrograph of the alveolar wall

Drawing of specimen 65

THE NEUROSENSORY SYSTEM

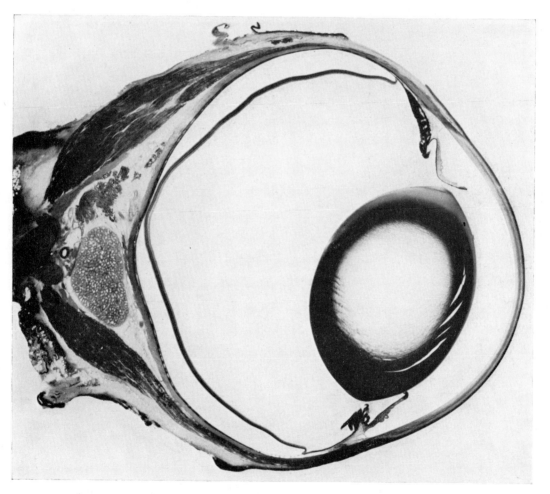

66. **Eye,** gross, V.S. (guinea pig), mag. 12x

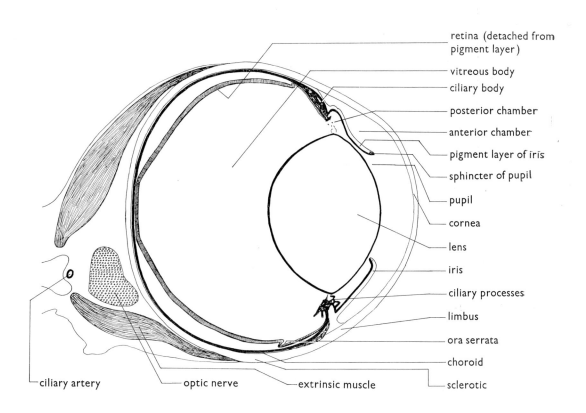

retina (detached from pigment layer)

vitreous body

ciliary body

posterior chamber

anterior chamber

pigment layer of iris

sphincter of pupil

pupil

cornea

lens

iris

ciliary processes

limbus

ora serrata

choroid

sclerotic

ciliary artery

optic nerve

extrinsic muscle

Drawing of specimen 66

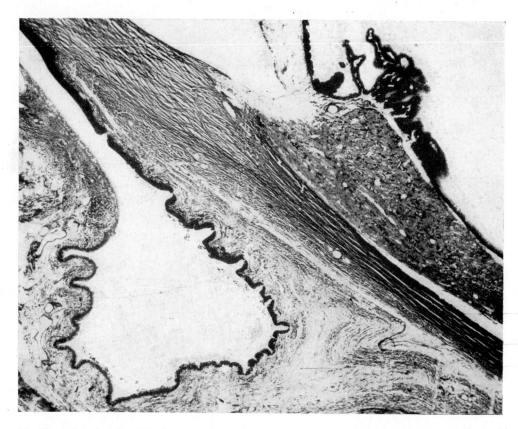

67. **Eye,** ciliary junction, T.S. (man), mag. 45x

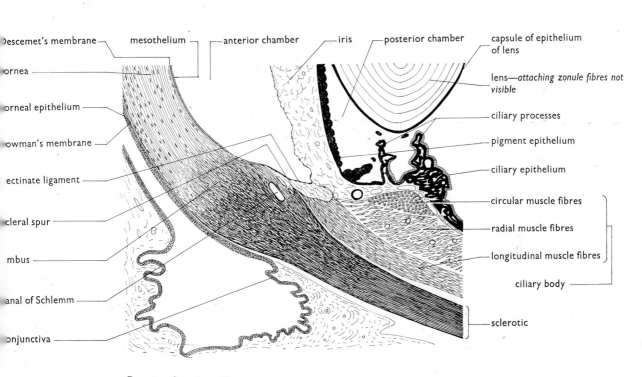

Descemet's membrane — mesothelium — anterior chamber — iris — posterior chamber — capsule of epithelium of lens

cornea —

corneal epithelium —

Bowman's membrane —

pectinate ligament —

scleral spur —

limbus —

canal of Schlemm —

conjunctiva —

lens—*attaching zonule fibres not visible*

ciliary processes

pigment epithelium

ciliary epithelium

circular muscle fibres

radial muscle fibres

longitudinal muscle fibres

ciliary body

sclerotic

Drawing of specimen 67

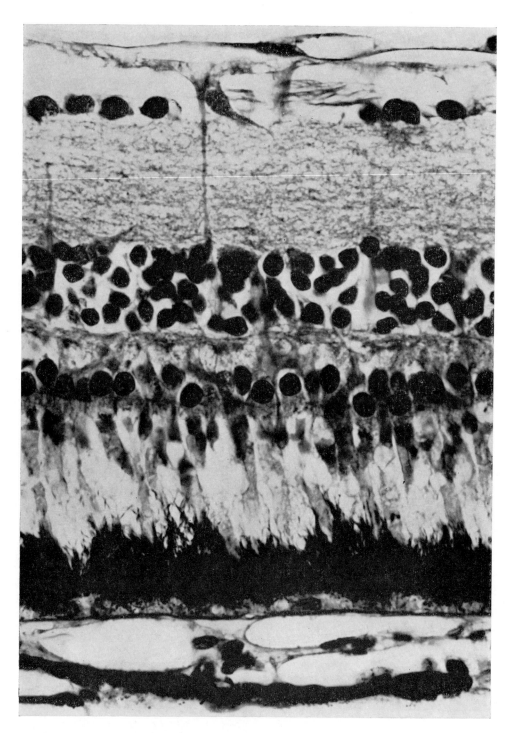

68. **Eye,** retina V.S. (man), mag. 950x

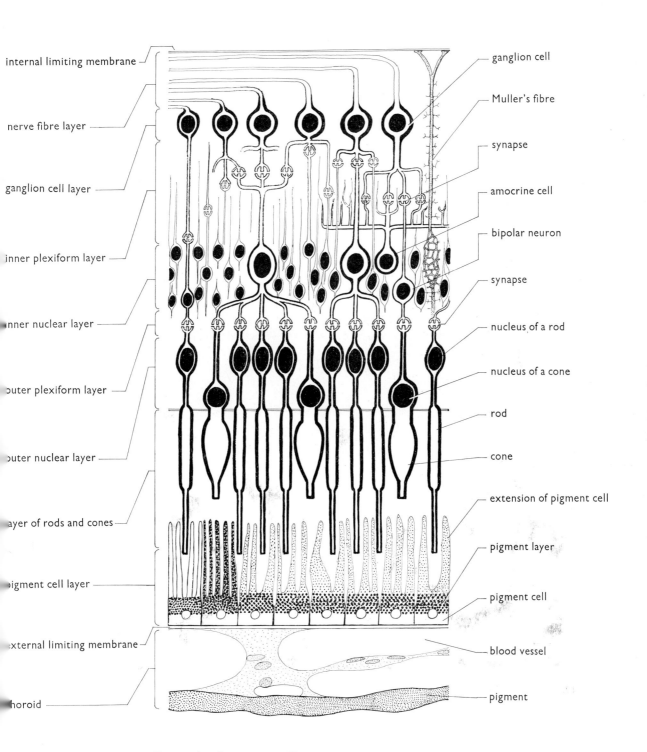

internal limiting membrane

nerve fibre layer

ganglion cell layer

inner plexiform layer

inner nuclear layer

outer plexiform layer

outer nuclear layer

layer of rods and cones

pigment cell layer

external limiting membrane

choroid

ganglion cell

Muller's fibre

synapse

amocrine cell

bipolar neuron

synapse

nucleus of a rod

nucleus of a cone

rod

cone

extension of pigment cell

pigment layer

pigment cell

blood vessel

pigment

Diagram based on specimen 68

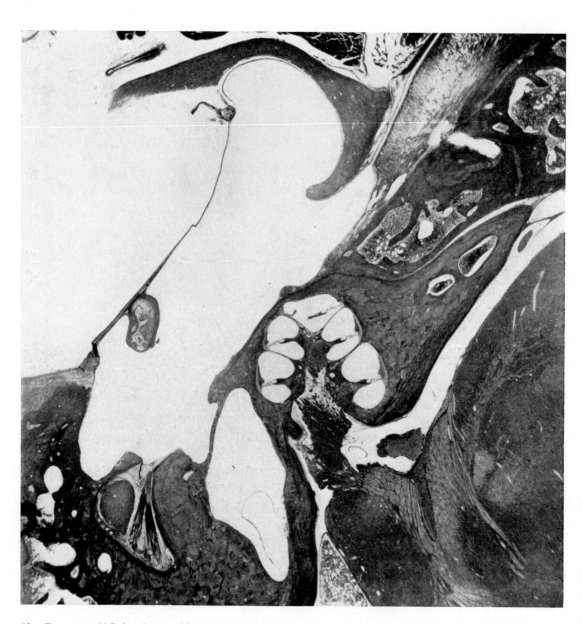

69. **Ear,** gross, H.S. (man), mag. 14x

front of head

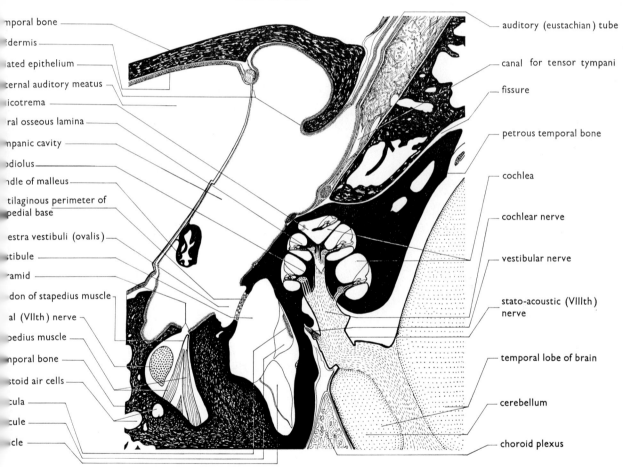

mporal bone

dermis

ated epithelium

ternal auditory meatus

icotrema

ral osseous lamina

mpanic cavity

diolus

dle of malleus

tilaginous perimeter of
edial base

estra vestibuli (ovalis)

stibule

ramid

don of stapedius muscle

al (VIIth) nerve

edius muscle

mporal bone

stoid air cells

cula

cule

cle

auditory (eustachian) tube

canal for tensor tympani

fissure

petrous temporal bone

cochlea

cochlear nerve

vestibular nerve

stato-acoustic (VIIIth)
nerve

temporal lobe of brain

cerebellum

choroid plexus

Drawing of specimen 69

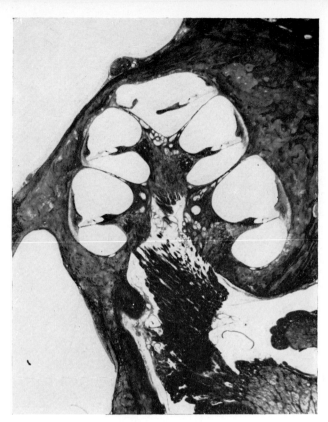

70. **Ear,** cochlea, H.S. (man), mag. 45x

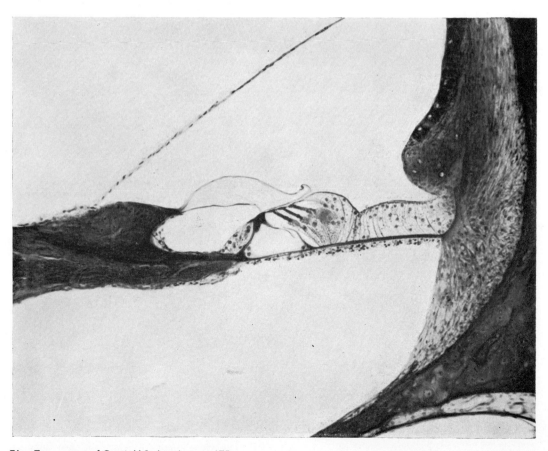

71. **Ear,** organ of Corti, V.S. (man), mag. 175x

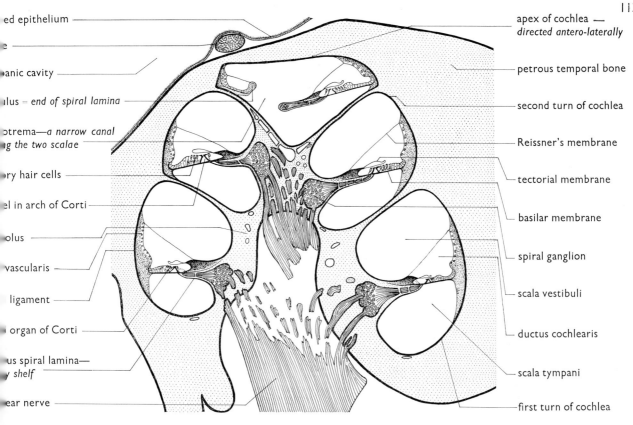

ed epithelium

anic cavity

ilus = end of spiral lamina

otrema—a narrow canal
ng the two scalae

ry hair cells

el in arch of Corti

olus

vascularis

ligament

organ of Corti

us spiral lamina—
shelf

ear nerve

apex of cochlea —
directed antero-laterally

petrous temporal bone

second turn of cochlea

Reissner's membrane

tectorial membrane

basilar membrane

spiral ganglion

scala vestibuli

ductus cochlearis

scala tympani

first turn of cochlea

Drawing of specimen 70

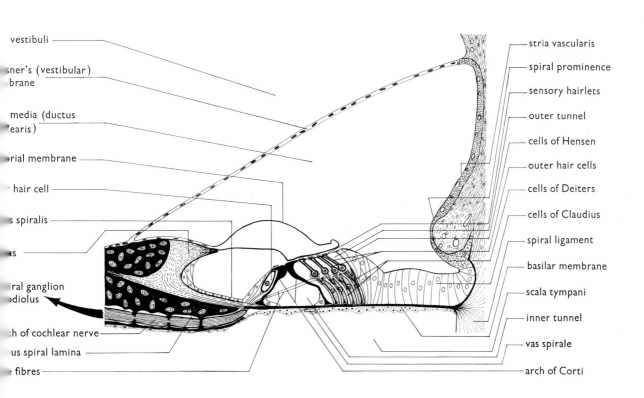

vestibuli

sner's (vestibular)
brane

media (ductus
earis)

rial membrane

hair cell

s spiralis

s

iral ganglion
diolus

h of cochlear nerve

us spiral lamina

fibres

stria vascularis

spiral prominence

sensory hairlets

outer tunnel

cells of Hensen

outer hair cells

cells of Deiters

cells of Claudius

spiral ligament

basilar membrane

scala tympani

inner tunnel

vas spirale

arch of Corti

Drawing of specimen 71

THE SPINAL CORD

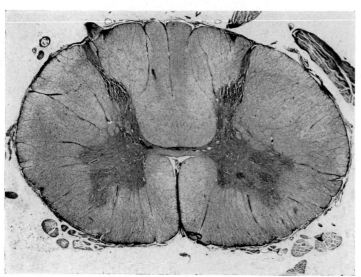

72. **Spinal cord,** cervical region, T.S. (man), mag. 7x

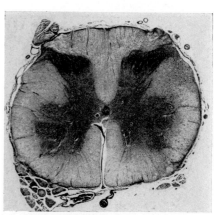

73. **Spinal cord,** thoracic region, T.S. (man), mag. 7x

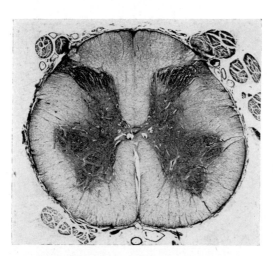

74. **Spinal cord,** lumbar region, T.S. (man), mag. 7x

75. **Spinal cord,** sacral region, T.S. (man), mag. 7x

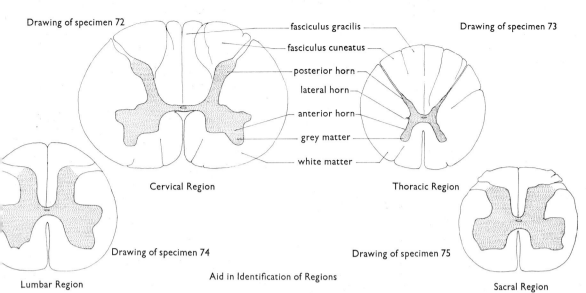

Drawing of specimen 72

fasciculus gracilis
fasciculus cuneatus
posterior horn
lateral horn
anterior horn
grey matter
white matter

Drawing of specimen 73

Cervical Region

Thoracic Region

Drawing of specimen 74

Drawing of specimen 75

Lumbar Region

Sacral Region

Aid in Identification of Regions

Region	Appearance in Cross Sections	White Matter	Grey Matter	Other Features
Cervical	large, oval	has greatest amount	posterior horns slender, anterior wide	fasciculus cuneatus as well as gracilis
Thoracic	small, round	considerable amount	posterior & anterior horns slender	lateral horn in some segments f. cuneatus in segments 1-4
Lumbar	larger than thoracic, anterior broader than posterior part	little	both horns wide	lateral horn in first two segments; fasciculus gracilis only
Sacral	small, slightly oval, almost surrounded by roots	very little	grey matter predominant; horns very wide	

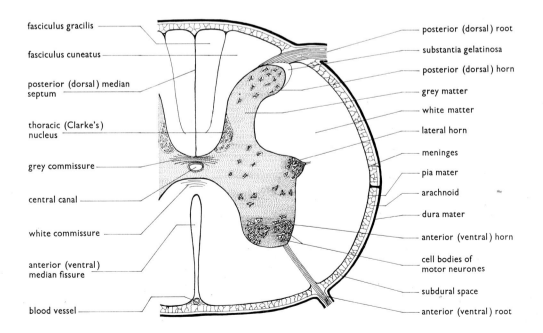

fasciculus gracilis
fasciculus cuneatus
posterior (dorsal) median septum
thoracic (Clarke's) nucleus
grey commissure
central canal
white commissure
anterior (ventral) median fissure
blood vessel

posterior (dorsal) root
substantia gelatinosa
posterior (dorsal) horn
grey matter
white matter
lateral horn
meninges
pia mater
arachnoid
dura mater
anterior (ventral) horn
cell bodies of motor neurones
subdural space
anterior (ventral) root

Diagram of General Plan of Spinal Cord

THE BRAIN

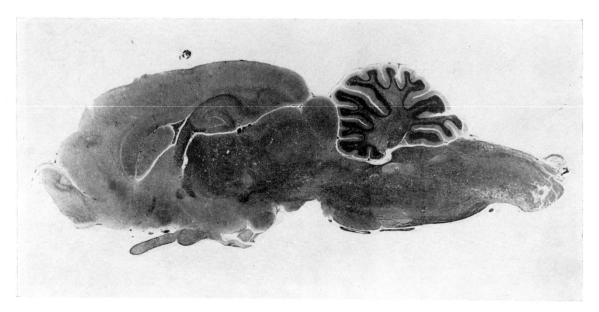

76. **Brain,** L.S. (guinea pig), mag. 3x

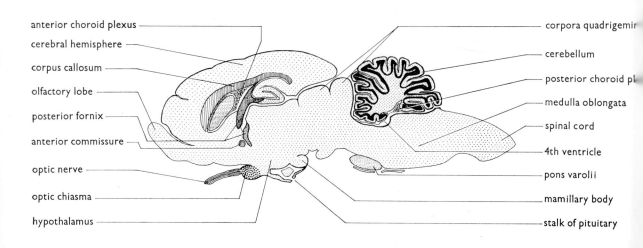

anterior choroid plexus
cerebral hemisphere
corpus callosum
olfactory lobe
posterior fornix
anterior commissure
optic nerve
optic chiasma
hypothalamus

corpora quadrigemin
cerebellum
posterior choroid pl
medulla oblongata
spinal cord
4th ventricle
pons varolii
mamillary body
stalk of pituitary

Drawing of specimen 76

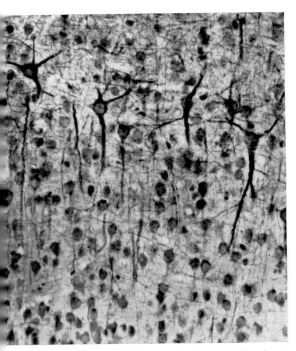

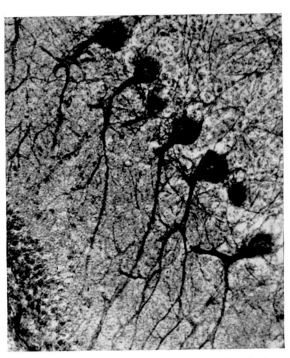

7. **Brain,** pyramidal cells from cerebral cortex (monkey), mag. 350x

78. **Brain,** Purkinje cells from cerebellum (monkey), mag. 260x

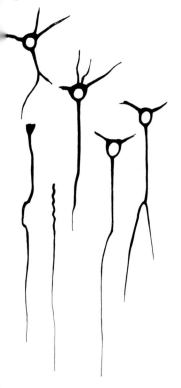

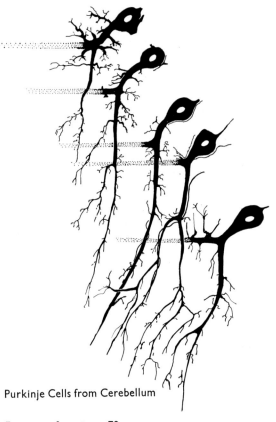

Pyramidal Cells from Cerebral Cortex

Drawing of specimen 77

Purkinje Cells from Cerebellum

Drawing of specimen 78

THE ENDOCRINE SYSTEM

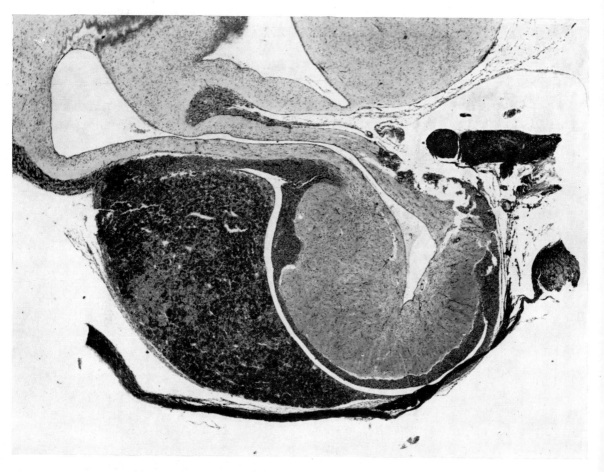

79. **Pituitary,** gross, L.S. (cat), mag. 32x

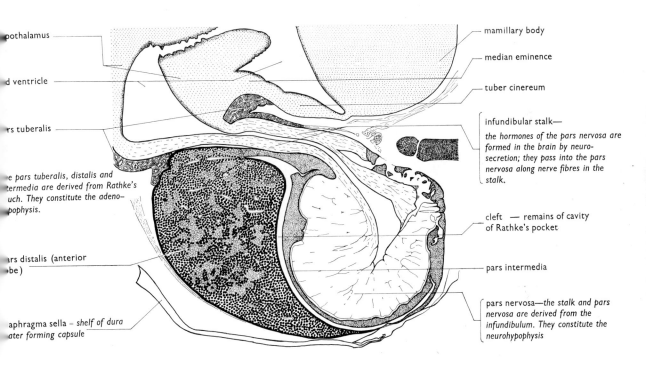

pothalamus

d ventricle

rs tuberalis

e pars tuberalis, distalis and
termedia are derived from Rathke's
uch. They constitute the adeno—
pophysis.

rs distalis (anterior
obe)

aphragma sella = shelf of dura
ater forming capsule

mamillary body

median eminence

tuber cinereum

infundibular stalk—
the hormones of the pars nervosa are
formed in the brain by neuro-
secretion; they pass into the pars
nervosa along nerve fibres in the
stalk.

cleft — remains of cavity
of Rathke's pocket

pars intermedia

pars nervosa—*the stalk and pars*
nervosa are derived from the
infundibulum. They constitute the
neurohypophysis

Drawing of specimen 79

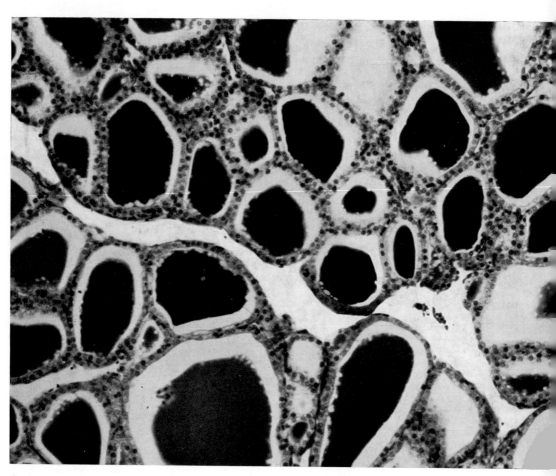

80. **Thyroid,** T.S. (monkey), mag. 380x

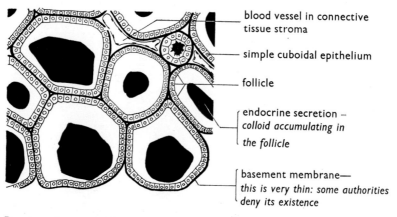

blood vessel in connective
tissue stroma

simple cuboidal epithelium

follicle

endocrine secretion =
colloid accumulating in
the follicle

basement membrane—
this is very thin: some authorities
deny its existence

Drawing of specimen 80

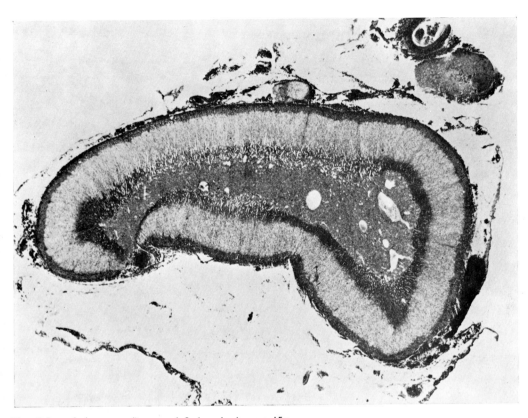

81. **Adrenal,** (suprarenal), gross, L.S. (monkey), mag. 15x

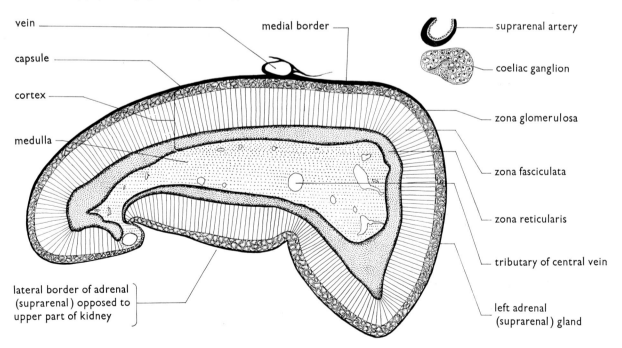

vein

capsule

cortex

medulla

medial border

lateral border of adrenal
(suprarenal) opposed to
upper part of kidney

suprarenal artery

coeliac ganglion

zona glomerulosa

zona fasciculata

zona reticularis

tributary of central vein

left adrenal
(suprarenal) gland

Drawing of specimen 81

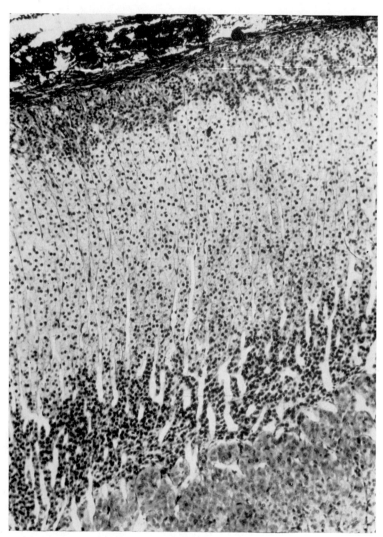

82. **Adrenal,** (suprarenal), T.S. (monkey), mag. 110x

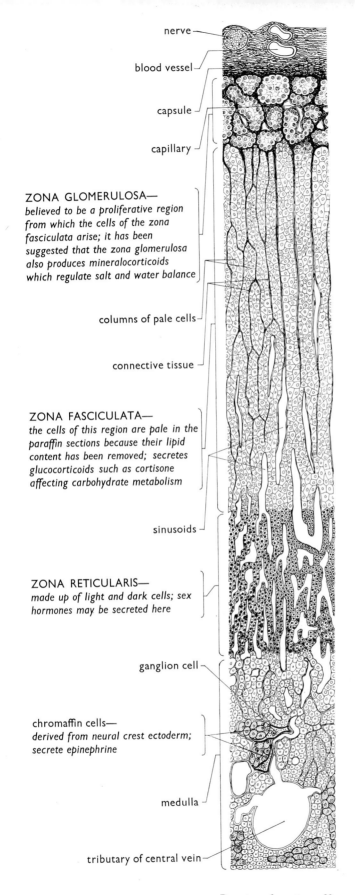

nerve

blood vessel

capsule

capillary

ZONA GLOMERULOSA—
believed to be a proliferative region from which the cells of the zona fasciculata arise; it has been suggested that the zona glomerulosa also produces mineralocorticoids which regulate salt and water balance

columns of pale cells

connective tissue

ZONA FASCICULATA—
the cells of this region are pale in the paraffin sections because their lipid content has been removed; secretes glucocorticoids such as cortisone affecting carbohydrate metabolism

sinusoids

ZONA RETICULARIS—
made up of light and dark cells; sex hormones may be secreted here

ganglion cell

chromaffin cells—
derived from neural crest ectoderm; secrete epinephrine

medulla

tributary of central vein

Drawing of specimen 82

THE CIRCULATORY SYSTEM

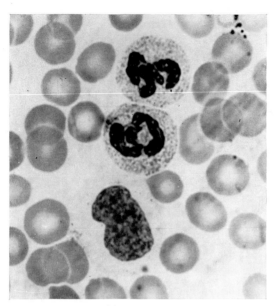

83. **Blood cells,** (man), mag. 2000x

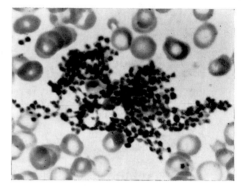

84. **Platelets,** (man), mag. 850x

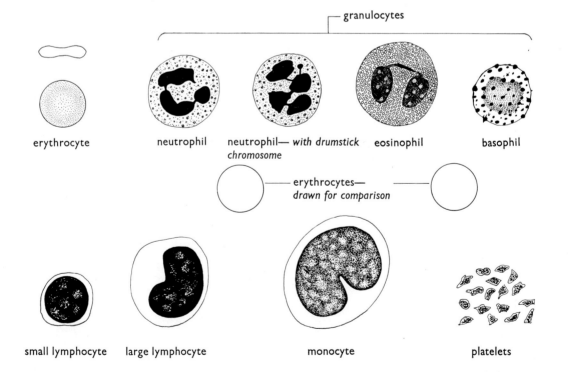

granulocytes

erythrocyte   neutrophil   neutrophil— *with drumstick* *chromosome*   eosinophil   basophil

erythrocytes— *drawn for comparison*

small lymphocyte   large lymphocyte   monocyte   platelets

Diagrams based on specimens 83 & 84

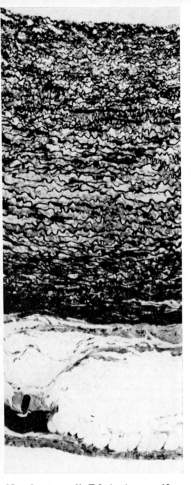

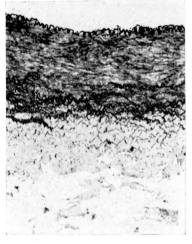

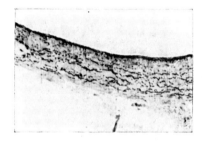

85. **Aorta wall,** T.S. (cat), mag. 60x   86. **Artery wall,** T.S. (cat), mag. 69x   87. **Vein wall,** T.S. (cat), mag. 60x

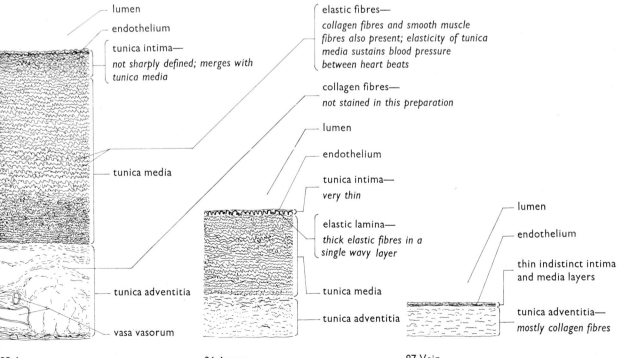

lumen

endothelium

tunica intima—
*not sharply defined; merges with
tunica media*

tunica media

tunica adventitia

vasa vasorum

elastic fibres—
*collagen fibres and smooth muscle
fibres also present; elasticity of tunica
media sustains blood pressure
between heart beats*

collagen fibres—
not stained in this preparation

lumen

endothelium

tunica intima—
very thin

elastic lamina—
*thick elastic fibres in a
single wavy layer*

tunica media

tunica adventitia

lumen

endothelium

thin indistinct intima
and media layers

tunica adventitia—
mostly collagen fibres

85 Aorta   86 Artery   87 Vein

ORGAN RELATIONSHIPS

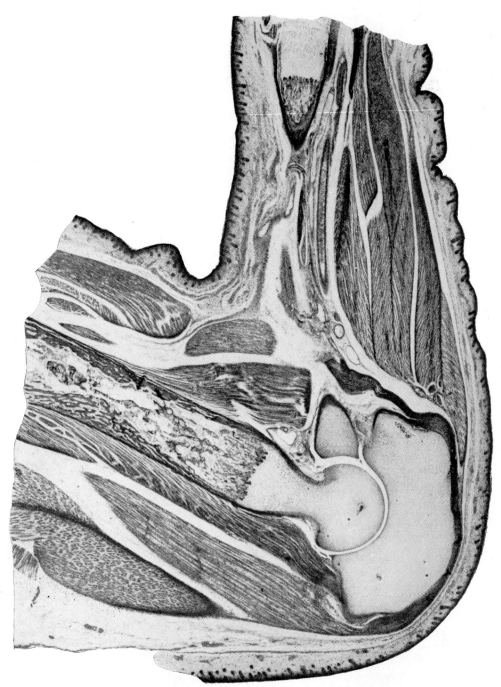

88. Elbow joint, foetal L.S. (rat) mag 12x

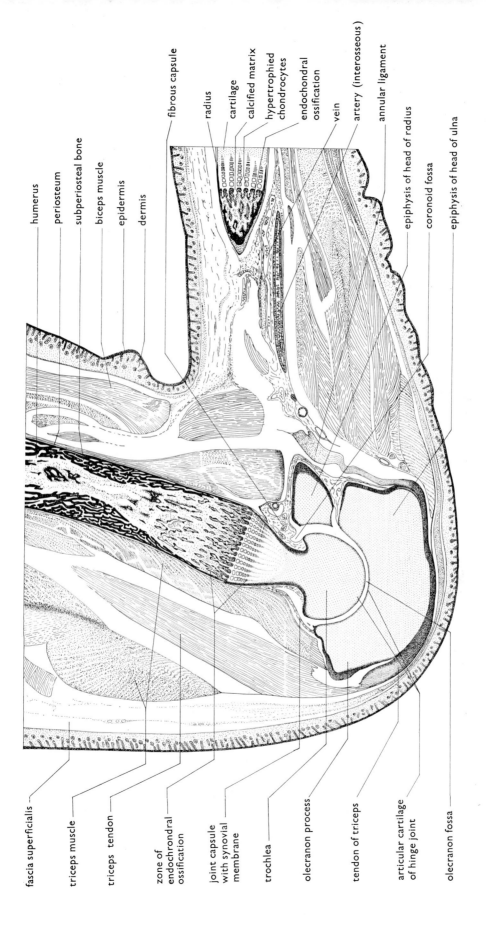

humerus

periosteum

subperiosteal bone

biceps muscle

epidermis

dermis

fibrous capsule

radius

cartilage

calcified matrix

hypertrophied chondrocytes

endochondral ossification

vein

artery (interosseous)

annular ligament

epiphysis of head of radius

coronoid fossa

epiphysis of head of ulna

fascia superficialis

triceps muscle

triceps tendon

zone of endochrondral ossification

joint capsule with synovial membrane

trochlea

olecranon process

tendon of triceps

articular cartilage of hinge joint

olecranon fossa

Drawing of specimen 88

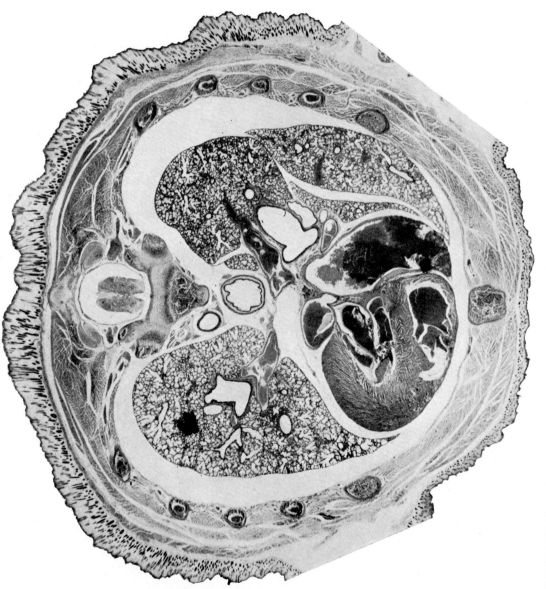

129

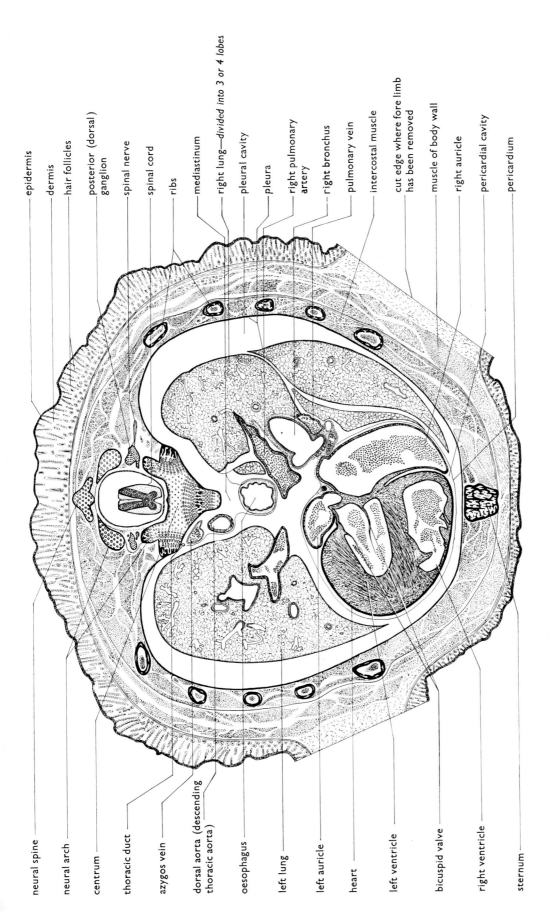

epidermis

dermis

hair follicles

posterior (dorsal) ganglion

spinal nerve

spinal cord

ribs

mediastinum

right lung—divided into 3 or 4 lobes

pleural cavity

pleura

right pulmonary artery

right bronchus

pulmonary vein

intercostal muscle

cut edge where fore limb has been removed

muscle of body wall

right auricle

pericardial cavity

pericardium

neural spine

neural arch

centrum

thoracic duct

azygos vein

dorsal aorta (descending thoracic aorta)

oesophagus

left lung

left auricle

heart

left ventricle

bicuspid valve

right ventricle

sternum

Drawing of specimen 89

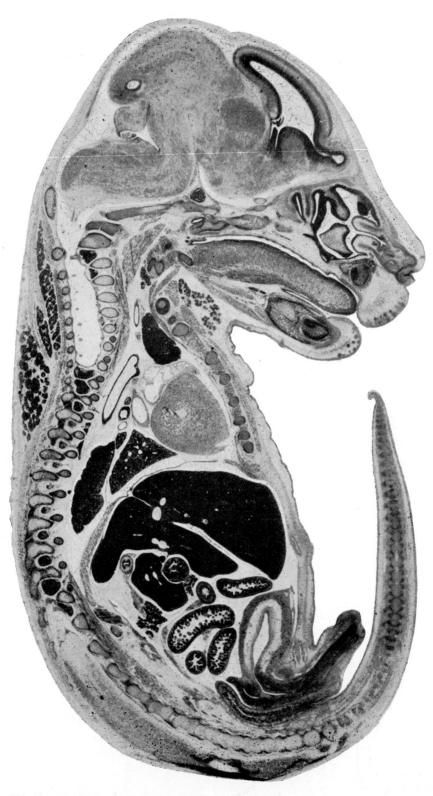

90. **Mouse embryo,** 10 days, L.S. mag. 12x

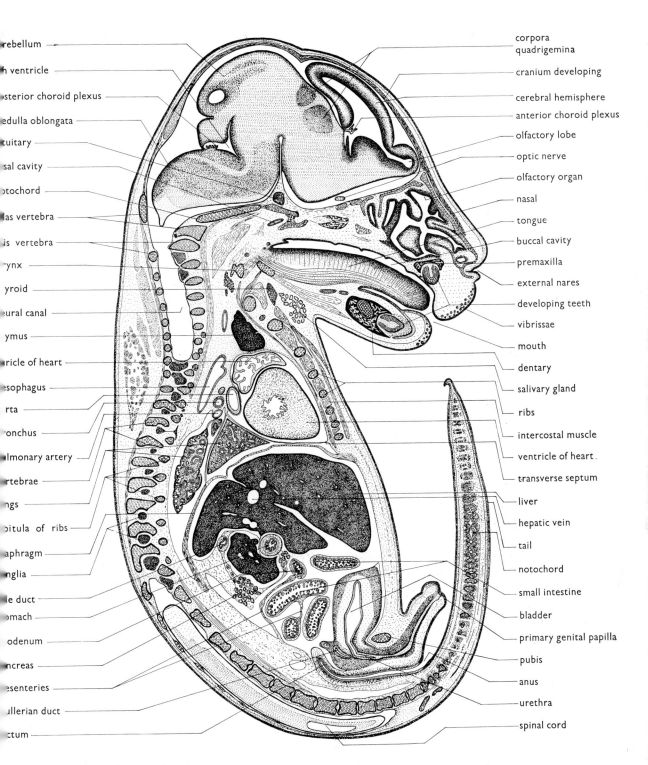

rebellum
h ventricle
sterior choroid plexus
edulla oblongata
tuitary
sal cavity
otochord
las vertebra
is vertebra
rynx
yroid
ural canal
ymus
ricle of heart
sophagus
rta
onchus
lmonary artery
rtebrae
ngs
pitula of ribs
aphragm
nglia
e duct
omach
odenum
ncreas
esenteries
ullerian duct
ctum

corpora quadrigemina
cranium developing
cerebral hemisphere
anterior choroid plexus
olfactory lobe
optic nerve
olfactory organ
nasal
tongue
buccal cavity
premaxilla
external nares
developing teeth
vibrissae
mouth
dentary
salivary gland
ribs
intercostal muscle
ventricle of heart.
transverse septum
liver
hepatic vein
tail
notochord
small intestine
bladder
primary genital papilla
pubis
anus
urethra
spinal cord

Drawing of specimen 90

MITOSIS

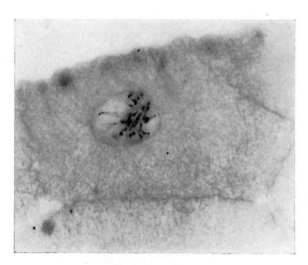

91 **Prophase** (whitefish blastula), mag. 1000x

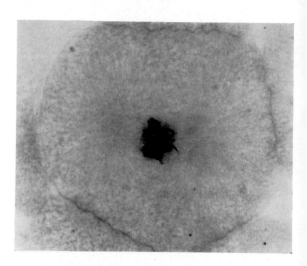

92. **Prometaphase,** (whitefish blastula), mag. 1000x

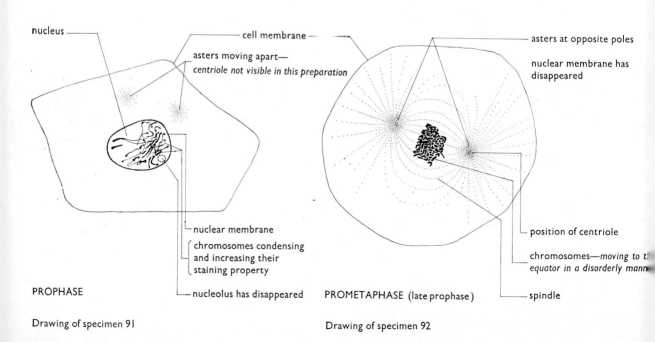

nucleus

cell membrane

asters moving apart—
centriole not visible in this preparation

asters at opposite poles

nuclear membrane has
disappeared

nuclear membrane

chromosomes condensing
and increasing their
staining property

nucleolus has disappeared

position of centriole

chromosomes—*moving to t*
equator in a disorderly mann

spindle

PROPHASE

PROMETAPHASE (late prophase)

Drawing of specimen 91

Drawing of specimen 92

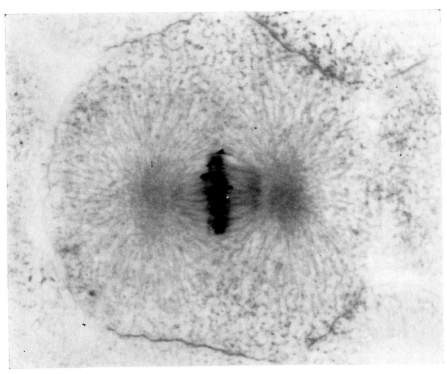

93. **Metaphase,** (whitefish blastula), mag. 1000x

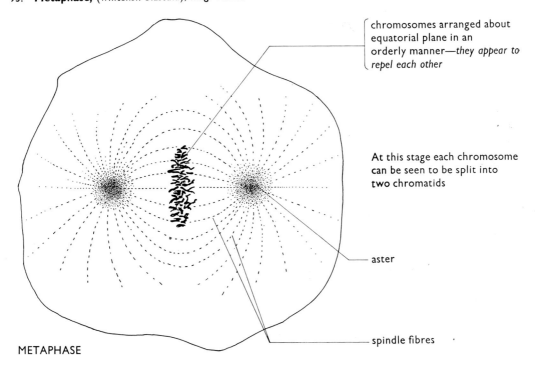

chromosomes arranged about equatorial plane in an orderly manner—*they appear to repel each other*

At this stage each chromosome can be seen to be split into **two** chromatids

aster

METAPHASE

spindle fibres

Drawing of specimen 93

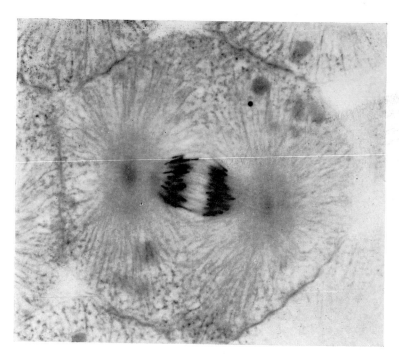

94. Anaphase, (whitefish blastula) mag. 1000x

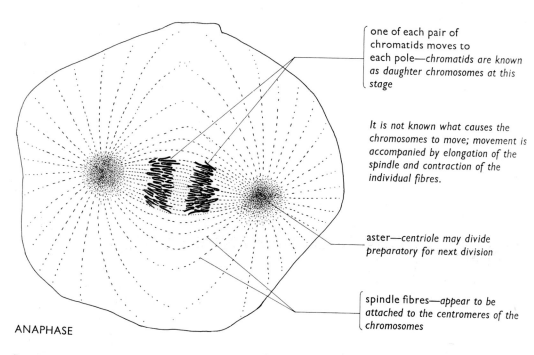

one of each pair of chromatids moves to each pole—*chromatids are known as daughter chromosomes at this stage*

It is not known what causes the chromosomes to move; movement is accompanied by elongation of the spindle and contraction of the individual fibres.

aster—*centriole may divide preparatory for next division*

spindle fibres—*appear to be attached to the centromeres of the chromosomes*

ANAPHASE

Drawing of specimen 94

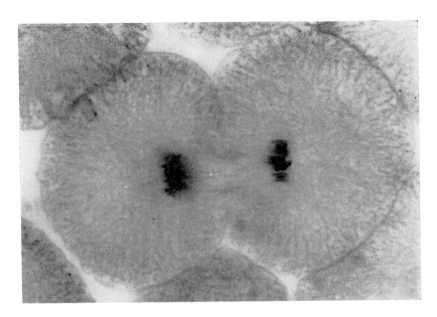

95. **Telophase,** (whitefish blastula), mag. 1000x

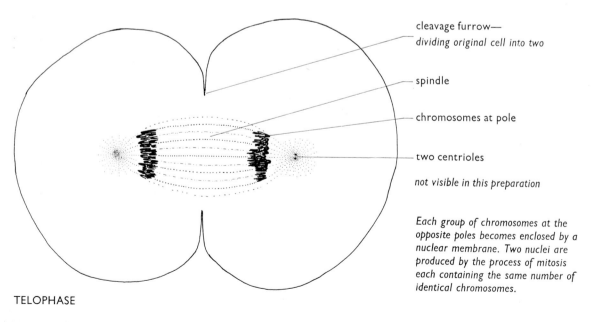

cleavage furrow—
dividing original cell into two

spindle

chromosomes at pole

two centrioles

not visible in this preparation

Each group of chromosomes at the opposite poles becomes enclosed by a nuclear membrane. Two nuclei are produced by the process of mitosis each containing the same number of identical chromosomes.

TELOPHASE

Drawing of specimen 95

Index